The Safe Approach

I0882813

The Safe Approach

Controlling Risk for Workers in the Helping Professions

Charles Ennis

Janet Douglas, MSW

Issues Press

Issues Press

An imprint of:
Idyll Arbor, 39129 264th Ave SE, Enumclaw, WA 98022
360-825-7797, www.IdyllArbor.com
Issues Press editor: Thomas M. Blaschko.

© Copyright 2007, Idyll Arbor, Inc. All rights reserved. No part of this book may be reproduced, stored in a retrieval system, or transcribed, in any form or by any means — electronic, mechanical, photocopying, recording, or otherwise — without the prior written permission of the publisher.

To the best of our knowledge, the information and recommendations of this book reflect currently accepted practice. Nevertheless, they cannot be considered absolute and universal. Recommendations for a particular person must be considered in light of the person's needs and condition. The author and publisher disclaim responsibility for any adverse effects resulting directly or indirectly from the suggested practices, from any undetected errors, or from the reader's misunderstanding of the text.

ISBN 1-930461-03-8
9781930461031

Library of Congress Cataloging-in-Publication Data

Cuhulain, Kerr, 1954-
The safe approach : controlling risk for workers in the helping professions / Charles Ennis, Janet Douglas.
p. ; cm.
Includes bibliographical references and index.
ISBN-13: 978-1-930461-03-1 (alk. paper)
ISBN-10: 1-930461-03-8 (alk. paper)
1. Social workers--Crimes against--Prevention. 2. Home health aides--Crimes against--Prevention. I. Douglas, Janet, 1959- II. Title.
[DNLM: 1. Allied Health Personnel--organization & administration. 2. Safety Management--methods. 3. Awareness. 4. Risk Assessment--methods. 5. Violence--prevention & control. WA 487.5.H4 C964s 2007]
HV40.35.C84 2007
363.11'93614--dc22

2006103554

Dedication

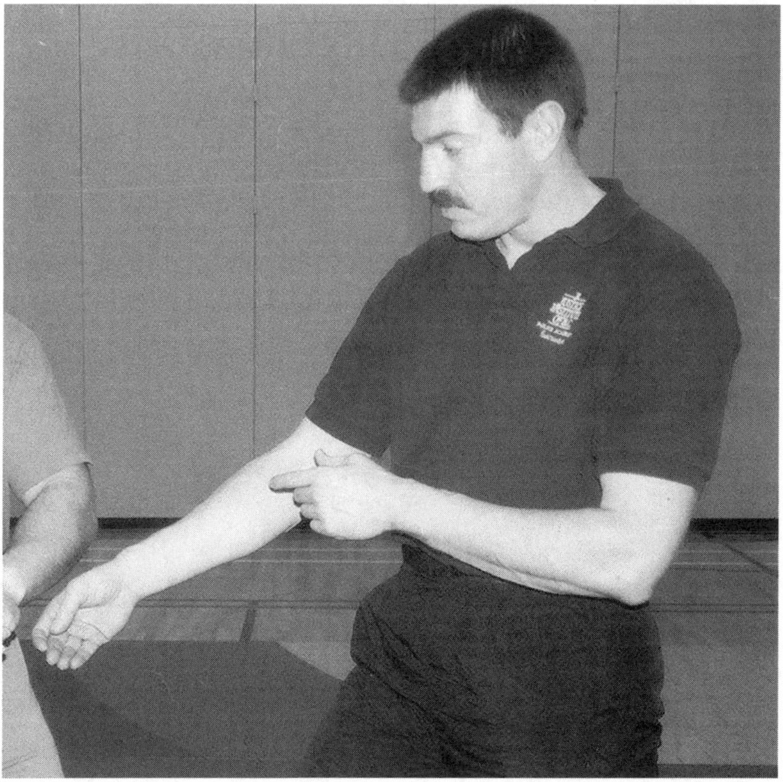

Photo by Val Ulyette

This book is dedicated to the memory of Charles' friend and partner Gil Puder, who died of cancer before this book was published. He will be missed.

Acknowledgements

The authors would like to thank Social Workers Bev Schultz and Val Ulyette of the Ministry of Children and Family Development, Vancouver Police Officer Gil Puder and West Vancouver Police Officer Eugene Knight for their help in the first photo session to illustrate this book. We'd also like to thank ECOMM police call taker Nicola Grice, Provincial Deputy Sheriff Michael Macro, designer Laurel Ennis, and Kamini Shaw from Black Bond Books for their help in the later photo sessions.

Photo Credits

Figures 1-2: Val Ulyette.

Figures 3-7: Laurel Ennis.

Illustrations for hold releases in Appendix B: Laurel Ennis.

Contents

Introduction

All of the helping professions, including social work and in-home health care, have undergone many changes in the past few decades. Violence against children and elders has increased. Society is taking a more serious look at the best interests of the child and the aging adult. Governments now put the needs of the client above those of the family.

Legislation is in place in most states and provinces that gives social workers the authority to remove children from their families to protect them from abuse and neglect. Health care workers are required, in most jurisdictions, to report suspicions of abuse. The public is reporting more cases every year, and the helping professions have taken on a "policing" element to ensure the safety of children and the elderly.

People have put forth many theories to help explain these changes in family violence: higher unemployment, drug and alcohol abuse, poverty, immigration, overpopulated urban centers, single parent families, and criminal activity. All of the above are factors that have an impact on the increased level of violence. As a result, not only do people working in the helping professions have to deal with a new set of social problems, they are also exposing themselves to increasing workplace violence.

The authors have almost fifty years combined experience in the fields of policing and child protection. We are aware first-hand of the dangers to which field workers are exposed. It is not our intent to convince you that violence toward workers in the helping professions is a problem; this has been well documented by other authors, and you probably know it already. What we hope to do is to show you how you can perform your job more safely.

Balancing the roles of helper and authority figure is a difficult task at the best of times, and can be confusing for the clients that we serve. An assessment of the likelihood of violence needs to include an examination of the client's reaction to your arrival. You must take into consideration the situation that you need to examine and the authoritative action you expect to take. Families will often welcome social workers or health care workers into their homes when they feel that the workers have something to offer them. They may be anticipating supportive services, financial assistance, or relief for their children. However, when a social worker decides to take protective action and remove the children from their home, parents often become hostile and violent. The threat of losing their children may cause them to go to any lengths to prevent that from happening. If the nurse decides that an involuntary admission to the hospital is the best way to protect mental health clients that are endangering their health, this can precipitate a violent reaction. Similar risks occur when action is required to protect an elderly adult. Introduce alcohol, drugs, or a propensity for violence, and the risk to the worker increases exponentially.

Families may have had negative experiences with social workers or others in the field of child protection. They may assume that the current situation will be a replay of a previous unpleasant encounter with the authorities, even if your intent is not to remove the children or do an involuntary apprehension. Media reports of field workers or their agencies mishandling cases can cause families to feel justified in questioning and even fighting against your authority. As well, adults in the family may be involved in criminal activity and fear being detected. These are dangers, but an awareness of all of the above, and attention to safety precautions, can help you carry out your job. At the same time your own safety will be enhanced.

We recognize that people in the helping professions work in many diverse communities, both urban and rural, with differing populations, cultures, and a wide range of levels of violence. We have tried to anticipate all possible scenarios, ranging from verbal threats and physical assault to attacks with firearms. Certain sections of the book may not be applicable to all workers, depending on their community and job description. Nevertheless, we feel that an awareness of the potential for all levels of violence should become an integral part of your routine.

What we will cover in this book are ways to prevent and reduce violence toward workers, using readily available tools and skills. We will walk you through the necessary steps to examine the risks in a situation to prepare for an episode of violence in the field. We will examine safety awareness. We will discuss the use of collateral information and the importance of file information. We will stress the need for ongoing safety assessment in a client's home. Finally, we will show you how to protect yourself should all else fail.

PART ONE

IDENTIFYING THE RISKS

1. The Reality

Reality is that which, when you stop believing in it, doesn't go away.

—Philip K. Dick

The goal of this book is to develop your safety awareness. This book will give you a new appreciation of the problems and risks involved in fieldwork. It will introduce new skills to help you deal with danger in the field. It will remind you of the skills you already have and use. This book outlines techniques designed to affect the way that you prepare for and react to violence directed against you. These are not theories. These are proven procedures, based on the experiences of workers who have experienced violence in the workplace.

We are going to start with an overview of the history of social work and health care work. After that we will be looking at some of the reasons for increasing violence and the reality of the dangers of the work you are doing.

The profession of social work has evolved over the past century, from its roots in the female dominated "friendly visitor" role of the late 1800s to its current place in society as providing government-mandated protection services. In the early 1900s, the rapid growth of urban centers made child and family poverty more visible. Middle class women were of great influence in the social work movement and began to work toward "rescuing" children from a life of poverty and crime. Their actions were mostly morally based. Back then, society afforded more protection to animals than to children, whom society still viewed as "family possessions." As a result, social work came to be viewed as a helping profession, supporting people and working toward the "greater good."

Reports of children being neglected, abused, and killed, often at the hands of parents, are becoming far too frequent. The American Humane Society reported that the number of child abuse reports in the US quadrupled from 669,000 in 1976 to 2,694,000 in 1991.[1] The National Child Abuse and Neglect Data System (NCANDS) reported that the rate of child abuse and neglect fatalities increased slightly over the last several years from 1.84 per 100,000 children in 2000 to 1.96 in 2001 and 1.98 in 2002.[2] NCANDS reported an estimated 1,400 child fatalities in 2002.[3] This translates to a rate of 1.98 per 100,000 children in the general population. NCANDS defines "child fatality" as the death of a child caused by an injury resulting from abuse or neglect, or where abuse or neglect were contributing factors.

These days, society no longer views child abuse and violence toward children as a "family" problem that we can overlook. Governmental agencies are taking greater responsibility for child welfare. They have created legislation assigning the responsibility of protecting children to agencies and organizations, and many nations have developed mandatory reporting laws. More and more social workers have been assigned investigative duties. Newhill[4] suggested that the risks involved with service delivery are linked to social control, as workers now have the authority to allow or deny access to resources. Anger at a social worker's actions may be an appropriate emotional response, but the problems arise when the person is unable to maintain self-control. "Social workers...are the only workers [with authority to remove children] who are expected regularly to visit the homes of violent people."[5]

A recent study by Stanley and Goddard found that "violence is an often successful way of controlling people, and allows persons to maintain control. When feeling threatened by child welfare workers, violence is often seen as a useful way to maintain control. When a protective worker becomes involved with a violent family it is illogical to believe that the protective worker will be immune from this violence."[6]

There are several reasons for increasing violence. One is that many countries have moved toward the deinstitutionalization of mental health clients into the community. Community resources for the mentally disordered have therefore had to expand to meet the needs of these clients. Thus mental health teams with outreach services have appeared. This, in turn, has increased the safety risks for nurses and workers who must go out into the community to deal with clients who have little insight into their illness, are noncompliant with medications, or who avoid contact with mental health authorities. Mental illness further complicates matters. This is not to suggest that all mentally ill persons are violent, but that certain risk factors and symptoms can enhance the probability of violence.[7]

Another reason for increasing violence is that the list of responsibilities for the helping professions now includes the allocation of scarce resources, the compulsory admission of mentally ill and mentally impaired people to hospitals, the investigation of domestic violence and cases of non-accidental injury to children, the removal of children from homes against the wishes of the parents, the compulsory removal of some elderly people from home to hospital, and the supervision of men and women in the community with a history of potential or actual violence, some with an associated mental disorders.[8] The role of aiding families and protecting children has taken on a new meaning. This has brought increased risk to social workers who are attempting to intervene with these families.

Criminal law defines assault as violence, real or implied, directed at another person. Violence, for the purposes of this book, can include anything from verbal threats to homicide. Verbal abuse, swearing, or threats can include those directed at the worker, the worker's family, or their agency. Intimidation by the client, both verbal and physical, is commonplace. Physical assaults can include grabbing, pushing, cornering, punching, scratching, or biting, and extend to sexual assault, choking, or body holds. Assaults with weapons range from the use of available household items to knives and firearms. Serious injury or death can and has occurred. As a worker it is important to remember that if an action has caused you to feel that someone has assaulted you, then you probably have been assaulted.

One of the obstacles in conducting our review of the literature is that there appear to be few studies on violence against workers in the helping professions. What follows is pretty much all that there is, but they are telling statistics indeed.

A London Boroughs' Training Committee studied cases of social workers killed at work between November 1, 1982 and April 28, 1983. They reported that "it is noteworthy that most of the social workers...killed have been field workers."[9]

In 1988 the BBC conducted a study that determined that "proportionately more social workers than police have been murdered on duty in England and Wales in the past three years."[10]

In 1993, according to the Bureau of Labor Statistics, 1,063 work-related homicides occurred in the United States, an increase from the 1992 number of 1,004. In the US in 1998, homicides dropped, accounting for 709 (12%) of the 6,026 work related fatalities, and were the second most common event next to fatalities resulting from motor vehicle accidents (1,431).[11]

An average of 1.7 million people were victims of violent crime while working or on duty in the United States, according to a report published by the Bureau of Justice Statistics (BJS), each year from 1993 through 1999. An estimated 1.3 million (75%) of these incidents were simple assaults, while an additional 19% were aggravated assaults. For the same time period, over 800 workplace homicides per year were recorded by the Bureau of Labor Statistics' Census of Fatal Occupational Injuries.[12]

The Washington State Attorney General's Department reported in February 1996 that, "Workplace violence is the third leading cause of all workplace fatalities. For women, homicide is the leading cause of death in the workplace, representing approximately 40% of the total number of workplace deaths."[13]

Several individuals and organizations have conducted sporadic research into violence toward social workers over the past two decades:

- In 1976 the Whitman study in the US determined that 43% of social and psychiatric workers had received threats from clients. Clients assaulted a further 24%.[14]
- A study in Wessex in 1979[15] found that 69% of social workers were victims of either assault or threats in the study period. Clients had assaulted 29% of the workers and had threatened a further 40% at least once. Clients assaulted 18% of the workers and had threatened a further 30% more than once. 12% of field workers had personal possessions damaged by clients. 42% of these incidents occurred in the client's home, 19% in an office and 11% in a car or ambulance while escorting the client to a hospital or residential establishment.
- A study by Berstein in 1981 in the US found that clients had assaulted 14% of all psychiatric and social workers and threatened 35% with violence.[16]
- In 1987 the Health Service Advisory Committee in the UK conducted a survey of 3,000 workers. They found that in the previous year 0.5% had sustained injuries requiring medical assistance and 11% had minor injuries requiring first aid. Clients had threatened 5% with a weapon and verbally threatened 18%.[17]
- In 1988 the British Crime Survey found that teachers, welfare workers, and nurses were three times more likely than the average employee to be verbally abused or threatened.[18]
- In Britain in 1989 the National Association of Local Government Offices conducted a three-month study of

violence against social service staff. They discovered that more than 33% of social services staff had experienced hostile behavior and that clients had physically assaulted 10%.[19]

- In the same year the British journal Community Care published a survey of 518 social workers. This survey showed that clients had physically attacked 68% and subjected 61% to minor assaults.[20]
- A DYFS study in New Jersey between July 1, 1992 and June 30, 1993 revealed 25 incidents of assault to workers.[21]
- In their study in rural Montana, Horejsi et al. (1994) found child protection social workers were most at risk, in that one in ten stated they had been pushed, shoved, or hit.[22]
- The American Occupational Safety and Health Administration reported that "in 2000, 48% of all non-fatal injuries from occupational assaults and violent acts occurred in health care and social services."[23]
- In a 2001 study in Canada by Macdonald and Sirotich, 63.5% of social workers in their random sample had been threatened with violence, and 28.6% had been assaulted.[24] However they also noted that "approximately 25% of respondents indicated that they did not report an incident of violence perpetrated against them by a client." Social workers cited lack of faith in management, feeling inadequate in their job,

and/or feeling it was a part of their job as their reasons for not reporting.[25]

In 1998 a large-scale study was conducted to examine violence in schools and the effect on school-based social workers. A questionnaire was distributed to 1200 school social workers, with a response rate of 52.8%. With respect to personal safety, one-third reported that they feared for their personal safety about once a month or more.[26] Significantly more social workers in inner-city schools (71%) reported fear for their personal safety than workers in urban (36%), suburban (37%) and rural (31%) schools.[27] Although social workers' personal experiences with serious forms of violence were relatively rare, 35% reported that they had been physically assaulted or physically threatened during the past year.[28] The assailants were identified as students in 77% of the cases and parents in 49%. In 11% of the cases the students involved were gang members. School social workers reported that they took a variety of precautions for their personal protection. Thirty-three percent reported that they left money at home, 24% avoided school after dark, and 11% avoided wearing certain styles of clothing or colors.

With respect to field safety, the research found that 74% of school social workers viewed home visits as potentially dangerous. However 82% indicated they conducted home visits for aggressive children. As well, the inner-city workers were more likely to view home visits as dangerous.[29] Almost 90% of the respondents endorsed more school violence training for social workers during graduate school.[30] "Training for personal safety is an area of great concern for social workers. More than half who reported fear also thought of leaving the profession because of worries of school violence. Formal education on personal safety could help social workers avoid or better contend with potentially harmful situations."[31]

A 1995 study by Newhill, specifically looking at violence towards social workers, suggested that social workers may be inadequately informed about the potential dangers of their job, or lack training to manage the risks.[32] Newhill's study stated that anecdotal evidence and limited data showed that violence, both physical and emotional, was increasing towards social workers.[33] Newhill also cited Schultz's social worker study in West Virginia, which revealed a lack of formal training in preventing or managing violent behavior.[34] Newhill's study of 1129 social workers found only 59% reported they had received training on working with violent and potentially violent clients and concluded that knowledge was important in reducing likelihood of violence.[35]

Although most of the data collected on violence towards social workers has been collected in institutional settings or from restricted samples, anecdotal evidence also suggests attacks are not uncommon in the human service field.[36]

Jayaratne, Croxton, and Mattison surveyed National Association of Social Workers members with master's degrees in social work who were in direct practice. The decision of whether behavior was abusive or violent was up to the respondent and therefore represents the "subjective experience of the respondent."[37] Social workers reported on not only their own experiences, but also whether they knew of a colleague who had experienced violence. The sample was broken down into public and private practice. The researchers found that 22.8% of agency workers reported being physically threatened. (These findings were supported by previous studies by Newhill in 1996.) They found that institutional mental health and protective services posed the most danger, and these workers also reported highest incidence of fear of assault (88.3%)[38]. Young workers (less than 45 years) also reported more incidents of physical threats than workers over age 45.

Jayaratne et al made a number of recommendations,[39] including:

- A need to address the issues of violence and encourage reporting and/or the institution of mandatory reporting policies.
- More training on safety, office safety, and home visits.
- That BSW and MSW programs include content on dealing with client violence and dealing with the personal impact of the violence.

The authors also noted that it is a societal responsibility to protect the workers who deal with difficult client and social problems.

The statistics speak for themselves. Clearly, violent clients are a reality with which social workers must cope.

◆ ◆ ◆

Next we want to address the attributes of social workers and health care workers toward violence in their professions. It might seem that these workers would be the first to speak out against violence and its prevention, but that does not seem to be the case. We think that safety needs to always be at the forefront. Yet safety and prevention in the field often get little attention from field workers. People in the helping professions are often so focused on trying to meet the needs of their clients that they forget to look out for themselves. It is often not until a worker or colleague has experienced an assault that it takes on a higher priority.

Social workers and nurses routinely conduct risk assessments on individuals and families. You need to conduct the same risk assessments where your own safety is involved. Proper planning and preparation can prevent many violent incidents from occurring and can enhance your ability to survive violent encounters.

Perhaps you are finding it difficult to believe that there is a lack of concern for personal safety, but here is what the studies have found.

Northwest National Life Insurance Company conducted a 1996 study of victims of workplace violence.

This study showed 58% of the victims of work place harassment, 43% of the victims of threats at work and 24% of the victims of work place assaults did not report the offence.[40] Victims may fear that their colleagues and supervisors will see them as less competent. In fact, some field workers seem to behave as if violence directed at them by the client is somehow acceptable.

As part of their 2002 review of child fatalities in Victoria, New Zealand, Stanley and Goddard examined both hostage theory and the Stockholm Syndrome as part of their analysis of social worker/client relationships where violence is present.[41] They determined that social workers may adopt defenses in response to the need for self-preservation and relief from severe stress. These behaviors may include:

- denial of threat
- rationalizing
- intellectualization of the situation
- identification with the aggressor
- black humor

Stanley and Goddard recorded an interview with a social worker regarding her "under recall of fearful situations." This social worker reported, "You have to keep suppressing a natural reaction so you can continue to work"; and "we normalize when we should be more apprehensive than we are. I don't know why we do this."[42]

The truth is that violence interferes with your ability to function effectively as a worker. Worse, allowing clients to behave violently towards you with no consequences for their violent action may be seen as giving these clients "permission" to engage in similar violent behavior towards you and your colleagues in future. In Britain in 1991 a Department of Health review of findings from child death inquiries "suggested that the level of protection given to children may be affected by violence to social work staff by parents."[43] Failure to deal with the problem carries a high cost. Reporting workplace violence is important in the management of potential violence.[44]

Let's look next at why dealing with violence is important. Assaults against workers in the helping professions can lead to reduced self-confidence and increased anxiety. Failure to deal with violence in the workplace can lead to costly litigation, negative publicity, absenteeism, lengthy sick leave, high staff turnover, reduced job satisfaction, and dwindling morale. The first step toward greater personal safety in the field is knowing where to draw the line. Scalera, in 1993, stated, "Social workers cannot effectively protect children or help families if they themselves are not safe. We can no longer view the threat of violence as part of the territory."[45] Violent behavior on the part of the client may be understandable, but it is never acceptable.

One major potential obstacle in assessing danger is the strong commitment by workers toward helping clients.[46] Field workers who have been assaulted at work may blame themselves rather than their client. Workers can feel they "did something wrong" or somehow failed in the therapeutic relationship when violence or treats occur. In 1977 Walkley, emphasizing the relationship between conflict and stress, commented on a typical reaction to social worker victimization: that the worker had somehow failed to function as a "good" social worker.[47] Walkley argued that watching a colleague "fail" somehow protects social workers from their own feelings of inadequacy or apprehension. Schwarz identified a similar tendency among social workers to "blame themselves, and each other, for the violence done to them."[48] Bibby observed that:

> Even when social workers have been aware of a client's history of violence, reports from those who have been attacked indicate a sense of shock and surprise that the event had actually happened. There seems to be a denial by social workers of the potential for violence against them and it has been suggested that this denial develops to prevent workers becoming overwhelmed by fear, and thus feeling ineffective and powerless.[49]

This book aims to replace such feelings with feelings of effectiveness and strength. We want to develop your safety awareness. Keeping yourself safe is an important first step in providing services to your clients. Field workers should constantly remind themselves of the following:[50]

- Social work and nursing can be hazardous occupations, demanding constant attention to your surroundings.
- The client's background, attitudes, motivation, willingness to reason, and propensity to violence may be quite different from your own.
- Using force to save yourself or the life of someone else may be necessary for you.
- Safety depends upon realistic and ongoing assessment of situations and practicing appropriate safety procedures.
- Preparation, planning, proper attitude, and fitness lead to greater personal safety.

Among field workers who have managed to survive violent attacks, more than one has admitted, "I was just lucky." Depending on luck is a poor substitute for taking constructive measures to prevent a violent encounter. The current state of knowledge of safety procedures makes your ability to stay safe in the field greater than ever. Yet more effort is likely to have gone into the counseling and support that a worker receives after an assault than that worker or that worker's agency devoted to worker safety before the assault.

Sometimes the safety training provided is inadequate or nonexistent. Sometimes field workers get assaulted because they failed to practice what they have been taught. In 1993 Tully, Kropf, and Price reported that in the state of Georgia only 41% of social workers had studied the clinical predictors of violent behavior. Only 32% had studied violence prevention and only 22% had been trained in safety measures for home visitations.[51] One study found that of those workers attacked, only 10% had received support from management following an incident of violence. 23% of those receiving no management support had left or seriously considered leaving social work.[52] A Canadian study showed that 24.1% of workers felt their agency would do nothing or that they would be blamed for the incident (13.8%).[53] 89.9% stated they reported violence with the intention of getting some support, and 82.6% made reports to ensure something would be done about the problem.[54]

Many agencies have no systematic record keeping system to record and monitor violence against workers. The British Labour Research Department (LRD) found that only 45% of the workplaces where actual violence had occurred had any system of monitoring violent incidents.[55] The LRD reported that only 31% of the workplaces had a management structure that identified an individual who had the overall responsibility for dealing with violence and abuse. As well, only 11% had taken any action over the issue, although 69% of the workplaces surveyed had experienced violence.[56] In 1986 Rowett observed that:

> Social work training courses take little account of the potential for violent incidents in the context of local authority social work. Moreover, because of the tendency of courses to “de-skill” generally,

> social work graduates tend to emerge from them either unable to transfer such skills as they have to practice (Parsloe 1979), or too unsure of themselves to operate independently for some years and yet they are placed in situations where their role confers on them enormous social power within months of qualification.[57]

A Canadian study in 1996 examined reporting by social workers in Ontario. Their definition of client violence included nonphysical behavior based on the recognition "that sustained verbal abuse and threat can inflict psychological and behavioral consequences on victims which can be as serious as those arising from physical assault."[58] This study found that the most common reason for not reporting an incident of violence was the perception that it was not serious enough to warrant reporting (68.9%).[59] Nearly as many social workers (65.5%) stated that they considered violence a part of the job.[60] This study concluded that "social workers need the necessary skills to predict and de-escalate violent situations, and need to be aware that under-reporting impacts the ability of management, policy makers and the like to assess the extent of the problem of violence towards social workers and plan accordingly.[61]

In 1995 Scalera studied incidents of assault among child welfare workers in New Jersey. He argued that while child welfare workers are responsible for protecting children and supporting families, they themselves need protection and support in order to fulfill this mandate.[62]

◆ ◆ ◆

Usually safety problems result from a combination of factors. Training may fail to accurately reflect reality. Perceptions of risks may not match the actual risks involved. A study by Carmel and Hunter in 1990 found that frequent training can improve the likelihood of avoiding assault.[63] Yet workers may receive no training in safety considerations at all. They are expected to pick up whatever they need to know on the job. Workers often believe incorrectly (according to some of the studies) that most people reach retirement without ever being threatened or assaulted. Day in and day out workers investigate so many situations where nothing happens that they become complacent. They may approach a situation casually, hastily, and with overconfidence because "nothing has ever happened before." They begin to assume that "nothing will ever happen."

And then it does.

2. Safety Awareness

The scars of others should teach us caution.

—Saint Jerome

When we first started doing safety training for social workers and public health nurses in 1996, there were concerns from the field administrators that the material being presented might cause fear in the workers, resulting in them never leaving the office. One of the first things that we do in our sessions is to ask the attendees to take a moment to write down past work situations where they found themselves in dangerous or violent situations. Many of them come up with personal accounts of risk and injury. In other words, these people have already experienced the dangers of the job. They are still doing their jobs, and their fear arises out of not knowing what to do about violent encounters with clients. They are attending classes like ours because they want strategies and techniques that allow them to overcome the fears and anxieties that they already have. If that is what you are looking for, this book will give you those strategies.

We are not advocating paranoia and fear about personal safety in this book. However, you can't make yourself safe unless you have a true appreciation of the risks involved. Only then can you adequately prepare for them. The best defense for any social worker is to be prepared before violence happens. Being prepared often makes it possible for you to avoid potential violence altogether. "Knowledge of one's own feelings of discomfort and fear about client hostility, the proper uses of professional authority, the indicators of escalating client anger and the techniques to de-escalate potential violence are critical to effective and safe field work."[64]

We are not talking about community relations here. Some concepts discussed in this book may seem severe, but we feel they are required for your safety. Realistic safety strategies can substantially reduce the number of incidents that escalate to the point of violence. The old adage "An ounce of prevention is worth a pound of cure" certainly applies here. Yet none of the strategies discussed in this book should be regarded as absolutes. There are no absolutes in safety. No two situations are exactly alike. The procedures in this book are options that you may add to your repertoire of skills. Safety is using your head.

Our approach to this is supported by Newhill in her critique of the literature on defining and predicting violent behavior: Newhill's study found that "certain client characteristics are associated with a higher probability of violent behavior."[65] Newhill wrote that she had been told by several social workers that their gut feeling told them a situation was becoming dangerous, but that they dismissed their feelings as silly or indicative of personal failure and did not ask for assistance.[66]

Your body will often react to impending danger before you become consciously aware of the risks. When suddenly confronted with violence, your body will automatically revert to an instinctive "fear-fight-flight mode." It has been our experience that workers often dismiss the physiological symptoms they are having when they begin to feel unsafe and attempt to continue their interview or assessment. They fail to trust their instincts. It is important for you to realize that our bodies react for a reason, and that we need to pay attention to our racing hearts and sweating palms. Your respiration rates will accelerate; your ability to distinguish time, colors, and distance will dwindle; your motor coordination will decrease; and your bowels and stomach will end up in knots. If you become aware that you are experiencing these symptoms you should begin looking for the cause. If you ignore them, you may end up being a victim of the client's violent outburst. When you are caught unaware you will instinctively revert to the way you have trained. If you have neither rehearsed nor planned a response, you will be left with a basic "startle response" which is rarely an appropriate response to a violent outburst.

Causes of Violence

Understanding the causes of violence is necessary in order to prepare yourself to meet the risks involved in the helping professions. A client may attack you out of panic, desperation, confusion, anger, fear, derangement, frustration, revenge, intoxication, hallucination, political zeal, or suicidal intentions. Kaplan and Wheeler put it this way:

> Robbed of power over his or her own life, an individual is at risk not only of feeling anger but of acting on it destructively to reclaim that power. Violence is a final way of restoring balance.[67]

Violence can occur anywhere. A London Boroughs' Training Committee study from 1 November 1982 to 28 April 1983 revealed that 59% of violence against social workers occurred in the worker's office. A further 10% occurred in the street, and 21% in the client's home.[68] In 1986 Brown, Bute, and Ford determined that over half the attacks on field workers occurred when they were undertaking statutory duties,[69] that is to say, doing things required of them by law. Let us look at some more common reasons why a client may react violently to your interventions:

Clients may fear loss of their personal liberty. The Wessex study found that deprivation of personal liberty was the source of 56% of all violence against social workers and public health nurses.[70] It is our experience that far more clients have criminal histories than many social workers realize and criminals are very sensitive to the potential for being incarcerated by authorities (which in their mind includes social workers and health care providers). One reason for this is because many social workers either do not have access to police records or do not avail themselves of this information. As investigators we are frequently asked to follow up on cases initiated by social workers earlier in the day. It never ceases to amaze us how many of these workers have unknowingly wandered into the residences of clients well known to police for violent activity. Often the reason that they've forwarded these files to us for follow up is because they encountered resistance or were threatened, assaulted, or run off of the property. If they had known in advance what they were walking into, they could have been better prepared and saved themselves a lot of trouble.

The client may be mentally disordered or have a drug dependency. Compulsory hospital admission of mentally disordered clients accounted for 30% of all violence reported in the Wessex study.[71] According to a Washington State study, the client's mental instability or intoxication due to alcohol and/or drugs was the cause of 26% of workplace attacks and 21% of workplace threats.[72] A paranoid client may perceive you as a threat. Psychotic clients may have worked you into one of their elaborate delusions. Elderly people may experience delirium or dementia as a result of infections, medical complications, or illness. One of the symptoms of this dementia may be violent behavior. Liquor and addictive substances adversely affect the judgment and restraint of addicted clients. Some mentally disordered people self-medicate with alcohol and/or non-prescription drugs. This often leads to violent outbursts.

Clients may fear that you are about to take their children away. The decision to remove children from a household to protect them from physical, sexual, or emotional abuse or neglect is a major source of violence against field workers. The Wessex study identified this as the source of 26% of all violence against workers.[73] Twenty-three of 55 reported critical incidents in British Columbia in 1995/96 reviewed by the authors involved the removal or recent removal of children from the family home.[74] The client's parenting abilities are being called into question, and he or she is at risk of losing his or her child. The client will probably experience feelings of anger, denial, and guilt. If the client is receiving financial assistance, the removal of the child may also reduce the client's income. This may anger clients, especially if they need the extra income to support an alcohol or drug habit.

The client may feel a loss of power or control. Attempts to advise or chastise clients accounted for 9% of all violence reported in the Wessex study, while intervening to protect a third party accounted for 3%.[75] The clients may have had negative experiences with authorities somewhere in their history. This may cause clients to resist your intervention. Some of your clients come from parts of society where resentment and defiance of authority are commonplace. At home, in school, in social circles, or in relationships, one of their principal means of communication is violence. If they feel that they are losing control of a situation, they may become verbally and physically abusive in an attempt to correct the imbalance of power that they perceive. Clients who are mentally disordered, intoxicated, or who have a propensity for violence may be totally absorbed in what they are doing. They may not immediately be aware of your arrival. Once they are, they may act impulsively.

Your actions may have provoked the client. Something about your actions or demeanor may have angered the client. Your manner may have been perceived by the client as condescending or critical.

Factors Involved

Males are responsible for most of the violence against those in positions of authority. For example: Of suspects that kill police officers, more than 96% are male. Most of these are less than thirty years of age.[76] British statistics show that males between sixteen and twenty-five years of age perpetrate most of the violent attacks.[77] This does not mean, however, that women aren't ever violent, as many social workers who have tried to apprehend a child from a mother can attest.

Many believe that female workers are at greater risk than male workers. However, crime statistics in Britain show that young males are the most vulnerable to physical attack[78] and that at least twice as many men as women suffer from assaults.[79] Males, however, are much less likely to report such assaults.[80] Males are often more vulnerable because they do not expect to be attacked as often as a female. This overconfidence can get them into difficulties.

The social worker has several disadvantages in violent situations. For example, workers are expected to investigate families involved in domestic violence. Any police officer can tell you that this is one of the most dangerous situations that they encounter. Yet most social workers have nowhere near the training and equipment that a police officer has when responding to such situations. A client can decide when, where, and whom to attack, on grounds that may be totally irrational and indiscriminate. On the other hand, moral and psychological considerations that inhibit quick, impulsive action usually influence the worker.

Clients know you won't make the first violent move. You may not want to use violence. You may find violence morally distasteful. Nevertheless, it is very likely that the client will not share your views. Faced with arrest, hospitalization, or with the removal of their children, clients may feel that they have nothing to lose. They may accept violence as a natural risk of their lifestyle. When they act, they are only thinking of themselves.

Studies of police confrontations in New York have shown that less than 1% of all shooting incidents occurred without warning.[81] The signs and clues were there, but the officers involved misunderstood what they observed. We can say the same of social workers and other helping professionals that work in the field. Most field workers probably could have emerged unscathed from violent encounters if:[82]

- They had understood the dynamics of violent confrontations.
- They had understood and properly evaluated the risks that they were facing.
- They had made contingency plans to deal with possible violent situations.
- They had known and, through practice, had mastered appropriate safety strategies.

In Rowett's book, *Violence in Social Work*, Steadman identified the following contextual variables in violent encounters with social workers: "the location and time, relationship between the [persons involved], relative size, strength, age, use of alcohol or drugs, presence of other people, and the reasons for the dispute."[83] Steadman concluded that:

> In general, the data...indicate some systematic associations between contextual factors and the seriousness of disputes. Violence is greatest when the dispute is outside the home, late at night, when

alcohol or drugs have been used by either party involved, in the presence of third parties, where strangers are involved and where the antagonist is larger and stronger than the respondent.[84]

In 1977 Bailey identified four ingredients in violent incidents involving social workers:[85]

1. **A state of arousal**. The client was upset or agitated for some reason, usually demonstrated by pre-assaultive behavior.
2. **A trigger**. The worker's actions or intended actions precipitated the violence.
3. **A weapon**. The client had access to a weapon or could reach the worker with his hands or feet.
4. **A target**. The worker was in a position that gave the client the opportunity to attack them.

Of these four indicators, the state of arousal and the weapon are the easiest to observe and do something about, as we will discuss in the rest of this chapter. The trigger is often unpredictable.

Pre-Assaultive Behavior

Usually there will be some clue or danger sign warning of violence. Something about the client's behavior will indicate his or her intent. Learning the body language of violent clients is essential to your safety. The states of arousal you need to watch out for are called pre-assaultive behavior, meaning that they are behaviors that clients use to work themselves into a state where they are able to perform violent acts or they are behaviors that are required before a violent attack can be made. You should always watch for displays of pre-assaultive behavior that will warn you of an impending attack. They include the following:

1. Pacing or restlessness.
2. Rapid breathing.
3. Grinding of teeth.
4. Clenched fists.
5. Sudden immobility or coiled postures indicating a readiness to strike.
6. Dilated pupils.
7. Flaring nostrils.
8. Sweating, especially when the temperature and the client's level of recent activity make perspiration unlikely.
9. Trembling of the client's hands and extremities.
10. Intent staring. The direction of the client's gaze may even indicate the client's intended target.
11. Bobbing and dipping movements. If the client begins to shift his weight, he may be adjusting his posture to allow himself to grab or strike.
12. Rapid mood swings.
13. Loud speech, especially if threatening.
14. Bizarre behavior.
15. Body language that does not match the client's verbal message.

If the client is exhibiting any or all of these cues, the situation may be escalating. It may be time to get out!

Weapons Awareness

Social workers are frequently asked to investigate reports of abuse and neglect. This sometimes brings them into contact with potentially violent people. Your safety as a fieldworker depends upon constant attention to your surroundings and realistic appraisal of the circumstances in which you find yourself. Yet most people entering the helping professions such as social work, nursing, or even police work have almost no conception of the reality of violence.

The only violence most of us see is the violence depicted on television. Serial TV greatly exaggerates the true nature of violence in the field in order to create drama and excitement. Unfortunately this TV action is what most people take to be reality. Nothing could be farther from the truth. Violent confrontations occur at close range, last only a few seconds, and are often in the dark.[86]

By carefully observing the client and your surroundings, you can deny the client access to things that could possibly be used as a weapon against you. By using basic safety techniques, you can reduce your vulnerability and make yourself a difficult target. Here are some suggestions to help you better assess the real violence that you may face.

The single most important thing that you must watch in the presence of clients is their hands. **WATCH THE HANDS.** Almost every weapon ever made was designed to be hand operated. The hands hold the weapons, and often the weapons can be the hands themselves. Try to keep the client's hands in sight, especially the area of his palms. If you cannot see the palm of the client's hand and if the client's fingers are not all straight, the client could very easily have something concealed there. Clients that conceal one of their hands behind their back may well have something dangerous held in that concealed hand.

Look around clients to see what is within their reach. Constantly be looking for things that could be used as a weapon. Many are obvious, such as knives, clubs, and firearms. Many are less obvious. For example, the most common stabbing weapon after the knife is the common screwdriver. Pens and pencils, scissors, letter openers, and bottles can all become stabbing weapons. A very common stabbing weapon used by substance abusers is a hypodermic syringe. A cup of hot coffee or tea can be used with devastating effects if the client flings the scalding liquid in your face. Rowett noted that when weapons were used in assaults against workers, the chosen object was what happened to be at hand, not a weapon that the client had brought into the area with the deliberate intent of being used in an assault.[87] Ask yourself: Is there anything within reach of the client that may be used against me if the client wanted to?

A very common weapon used for self-defense nowadays is an aerosol such as Mace or oleoresin capsicum (OC, otherwise known as "pepper spray"). Pepper spray is sold over the counter as a dog or bear repellent or as a self-defense device, although in some countries federal, state, and/or local laws may prohibit its use or sale. It comes in a small aerosol container: small enough that most can be quite easily concealed in a person's hand. One sprays it in the attacker's eyes, causing the attacker intense pain and irritation but no permanent damage. The problem is that since its introduction, many people have purchased it to use as a weapon. The worker should be suspicious of any small aerosol containers within the client's reach. We'll talk about whether you should carry it later on.

We don't want you to become obsessed or overly preoccupied with safety. However, you will never be safe if you ignore the realities of modern social work. Safety is a matter of ongoing assessment of your surroundings and making timely decisions based on that assessment. Safety is a matter of constantly reviewing your actions to learn from your mistakes. You must develop safety awareness.

Chapter 2 Summary

- The best defense is being prepared.
- Safety is a state of mind.
- Acknowledge your feelings and reactions.
- Overconfidence is dangerous.
- Violence rarely occurs without warning.
- Realistically assess the risks involved.
- Watch the hands.
- Look for weapons within reach of the client.
- Don’t get too close: Allow an adequate reaction gap.

3. Attitude

Human beings, by changing the inner attitudes of their minds, can change the outer aspects of their lives.

—William James, US Pragmatist, philosopher and psychologist (1842 - 1910)

Safety is a state of mind. Safety is about understanding yourself. Your attitude is one of the most important aspects that can affect your safety. Adopting the attitude that "it will never happen to me" is as foolish as it is reckless. Safety is about 75% attitude, 15% skill, 5% physical, and only 5% luck.[88] Police defensive tactics instructor Tony Blauer puts it this way:

> ...one must first appreciate the three-dimensional integrity of the behavioral system. Simply put: How you think (psychological) determines how you feel (emotional). How you think and feel affects what you do (behavioral). Naturally, how you think, feel and behave will affect your choices (strategy) and your performance [tactics]...The truth is that your thoughts and

behavior will either enhance or encumber your tactical options. The mind navigates the body.[89]

One of the biggest obstacles to safety is overconfidence. Some workers seem to rely on no more than their air of authority to see them through. This is what Blauer calls "presumed compliance."[90] In Cosner's 1989 study of worker assaults in the state of Pennsylvania, respondents said that errors in the use of authority were frequently present in violent situations reported to the study.[91] The vast majority of clients are not intimidated just because you are a person in authority; in fact, this may even impel them to act.

We have experienced situations where social workers have attended homes and attempted to use their authority to establish a starting ground for the interview. One incident involved a worker who introduced himself to the client by flashing his identification in her face and then proceeding to quote the relevant section of the legislation that gave him the authority to investigate her situation. The client was intoxicated, as were the other adults in the home. The situation escalated immediately, and the social worker was at risk of being assaulted had the police not intervened. Had the worker taken the time to assess the situation and adopt a more low-key approach, this situation may not have occurred.

As we mentioned in chapter two, your actions can either provoke or calm the client. Violence can result if your actions or demeanor anger the client. Your manner may be perceived by the client as condescending or critical. It is important to be aware of the cultural background of the client. Expressions and gestures that are considered innocuous in your culture may be considered insults in another. Recognition of the diversity of the clients you work with, and training in cultural competencies, can assist you in dealing more effectively with cultural differences and avoiding misinterpretations. By using appropriate interview techniques you can usually calm a volatile situation and prevent it from escalating to the point of violence. By dressing, speaking, and gesturing appropriately you can avoid supplying verbal or visual triggers that may arouse the client's anger.

The distinction between power and authority is made by Weber in his discussions of bureaucracies and organizations. Weber differentiates between power and authority this way: Power is defined as "the probability that one actor within a social relationship will be in a position to carry out his own will despite resistance,"[92] while authority is "the probability that certain specific commands from a given source will be obeyed by a given group of persons."[93] Legal authority, as defined by Weber, is based on a belief in the supremacy of the law. It assumes the existence of a formally established body of norms and conduct organized for the rational pursuit of specified goals.[94] As workers, reliance on authority needs to be tempered by the client's perceptions of your position.

Collaborative actions are necessary when the social worker and client must work together towards a common goal. Being aware of their position and working together to form solutions assists clients to empower themselves and develop a sense of control.

Social and health care workers should strive to develop a level of comfort with their authority, position, and skills. The use of self-examination, increasing your own self-awareness, and recognizing your strengths and weaknesses can assist you in being safe in the field. Overconfidence and misuse of authority can be threatening to clients and affect your ability to establish a safe and trusting relationship.

Bibby, in her book, *Personal Safety for Social Workers*, suggests that a defensive approach to safety is disadvantageous because "it can lead to people failing to recognize opportunities to calm situations because they are busy planning their defense."[95] The strategies and techniques that we are presenting here do not call upon you to be preoccupied with safety to the detriment of your primary goals. On the contrary, the effective use of de-escalating or calming techniques is an integral part of this system. We are advocating safety awareness, not preoccupation. We are advocating a balanced approach. If you are so intent on trying to calm a person that you are overlooking obvious pre-assaultive behavior, you are not safe. The techniques that we are presenting here should become habitual and, as such, will not distract you from your fieldwork.

Be clear on your agenda before you leave the office. What is the minimum that you need to accomplish on the call? If your plan is to remove children from their home, or hospitalize a mentally ill client, then enlisting the assistance of police from the onset may make safety sense. However, if your minimum goal is to see that a family has food, or that an elderly adult has received a health visit, then your chances of accomplishing this safely without assistance are greater.

Remember: authoritative action by social workers often requires someone to give up something against their free will, be it their children in a protection matter, or their freedom in a mental health hospitalization. This is rarely going to happen voluntarily, and you should not attempt negotiations without police assistance.

Additional Preparatory Safety Measures

Backup workers: When at all possible, try to avoid going alone in field investigations. There is greater security in numbers. Always plan to attend a client's residence with a colleague. One field worker can act as the primary interviewer and investigator; the other acts as a backup worker. The backup worker can keep an eye on the situation, allowing the primary worker to concentrate on the job at hand. Although this is no guarantee of safety, an extra pair of eyes may discourage a client from acting rashly.

Dress and Presentation: One often overlooked but important safety measure is a worker's choice of clothing. Although we recognize that looking professional is important, there are ways to achieve this and at the same time be practical. For females, wearing flat shoes instead of high heels makes leaving a residence in a hurry less dangerous, especially if you are carrying a child in your arms. Avoid earrings that can be pulled or torn off. Long hair is an obvious target for someone to grab onto. A client can use heavy necklaces to strangle you. They can grab the straps of purses. Avoid carrying a purse; instead try to put as much in your pockets as necessary, or carry it all in a briefcase if need be. A waist pack or fanny bag is another possibility if it meets the dress requirements of your organization. The mental picture of a worker in high heels, with a purse slung over her shoulder, a briefcase in one hand, and a cellular phone in the other does not make much safety sense. As for males, it is best to save neckties for court. If they must be worn, invest in the clip-on style.

A final word about clothing: more than once, we have had low-income clients tell us that they had difficulty dealing with workers whose outfits cost more than they would receive for income for an entire month. This does not bode well for establishing a good working relationship, which in itself can enhance safety. It is a good idea to leave the jewelry at home.

Limiting Accessories and Baggage: Try to limit the number of things that you bring into the client's residence. You won't need more than your agency identification, your driver's license, and a single credit card or a small quantity of cash in case you are a long way from the office and must fill up your car or purchase a meal. Leave your wallet or purse with all of the rest of your money and cards at home or back at the office.

Don't spread around the items that you do carry. You do not want to have to waste a lot of valuable time retrieving them if you decide that you need to leave in a hurry. Try to avoid bringing in paperwork from the office. A general rule of thumb is don't bring in anything that you wouldn't want the client to read. More than one worker has been caught off guard when the client found paperwork inadvertently left behind or when the client read paperwork left lying around by the worker while the worker was distracted. Such reports may contain material that could anger the client and precipitate a violent response.

Communication: Don't develop the attitude that you are a lone wolf. Keep in communication with other members of your team. If possible, take some form of communication, such as a cellular phone, with you when you go to conduct field investigations. Make sure the batteries are charged and functioning before you leave the office. Take a spare battery. Recognize that in some areas there is no cellular phone communication available. If this is a concern in your area, you need to discuss alternative methods of communication, such as two-way radios, with your organization.

Even if you do have some form of communication such as a radio or cellular phone, always call and tell your office where you will be. ALWAYS tell the office what time you expect to call them back. If you do not call in by this check in time, your supervisor should then check on you to see if you are safe. If they can't contact you, they can send for assistance. Many offices have established sign-out boards to help monitor this situation. A code word or phrase that you can use as a "distress" signal is also useful. You can use it over the phone to tell your co-workers you are in danger. This way you can call your agency and get them to send assistance without the client being aware of what you are up to.

If you do have to call the local law enforcement agency for assistance, you need to know certain things that may speed up their response:

All calls to 911 or emergency lines for police are prioritized in categories to determine how quickly they will require a police unit to respond. Top priority calls are those that are in progress, involving violence or considerable risks. Examples include robberies, burglaries in progress, and domestic assaults in progress. Dispatchers will send police to these calls as soon as possible. At the other end of the spectrum are low priority calls in which the suspect has left, the risk is small, and the police that attend will simply be taking a report. If you must call for police assistance, make sure that you pass on ***all*** of the information that you have to the operator taking the call. If you have come across a domestic fight or fear an imminent attack by a client, tell the dispatcher this. If they do not understand that the incident is in progress, they may not classify it high enough to get you a timely response. If you do not have 911 in your community, ensure that you have memorized the emergency number, or call the Operator.

Always tell the police what you look like and what vehicle you are driving. This will help the officers to locate you. It may save them valuable seconds if they arrive on the scene and find you struggling with a client. They will immediately know which of you is the victim and take appropriate action.

Having the right attitude and recognizing pre-assaultive cues are only part of the safety equation. In the next chapter we will look at the planning and preparation that can enhance safety.

Chapter Three Summary

- Don’t rely on your air of authority to maintain control of a situation.
- Avoid being condescending or critical.
- Be aware of how cultural differences may affect your interactions.
- Be clear on your agenda before you leave the office.
- Take a backup worker.
- Dress appropriately.
- Take only what you need.
- Take some form of communications (a cellular phone, radio, etc).
- Make sure all batteries are charged.
- Make sure your vehicle is serviceable.
- Tell your office where you will be and give them a check-in time.
- If calling police, tell them where you are, what you look like, and how urgently you need them.

4. Preparation, Information Gathering

Violence does not and cannot exist by itself.
—Alexander Solzhenitsyn

Many field workers fail to consider that there is a great deal about ***any*** situation and the people involved in it that they do not and ***cannot*** know. They make presumptions based on experience or the history of a case, then suddenly find themselves confronting a situation for which they have not prepared. "Predictions of immediate or future violence are no more than relative judgments of potential risk(s) based on the practitioner's clinical experience and knowledge of the literature."[96] Cosner observed that any home that is unsafe for a child is also potentially unsafe for the professional social worker.[97]

From a safety standpoint, investigations must begin before the worker even leaves the office. The first thing required is an adequate risk assessment. For this you need to get as much background information as possible before you meet with a client in your office or attend a client's residence to begin an investigation. People who use violence against social workers often have a documented history of violence. For example, more than 60% of suspects who shoot at police have been arrested before on criminal charges, about 40% of these for violent crimes.[98]

Prior to attending at the client's residence you need to examine the history connected to this residence as documented by your own and other agencies and look for the following:

- Mention of firearms and other weapons.
- Documented violence, both domestic and toward people in authority.
- Affiliation with organized crime, gangs, militias, or extremist cults.
- Mental illness, especially indications of aggressive or suicidal behavior.
- Substance abuse.

A common scenario is a complaint filed by the non-offending parent. Social workers may investigate concerns of abuse or neglect without bothering to check on the background of the offender. Their investigation would include attending the home, speaking with the alleged offender, and deciding for the child. However, it has been our experience that contacting police before approaching the offender often provides significant information affecting both your safety and the safety of the child. It is common for police to know the party, including information regarding the individual's history of violence, ownership of weapons, or substance abuse. The party may be wanted on warrants or restrained by bail or probation orders listed in the police computer system. A field worker attending a home with just the information obtained from the complaint and the agency records would have no idea that he or she was walking into a potentially dangerous situation. Checking all possible sources of information before attending at a residence to commence an investigation is very important.

When deciding to attend a family's home, you must first examine your agency's history and relationship with them. Is this a family on your own caseload? Have you met them before, or are you a relief worker with no established relationship? Is the nature of your visit significantly different from previous visits? For example, you may be faced with having to conduct a protective investigation when you have previously been involved in a supportive role. This change of purpose can influence the reaction of the family, and increase the threats to your safety. Rowett noted that 60% of clients involved in assaultive behavior had existing relationships with their workers that were of at least six months duration.[99] It is therefore important not to assume that initial investigations pose a greater threat to worker safety. When working temporarily in an office, you will be at a disadvantage. To assess your safety you will be relying on written notes and information from colleagues, which are often not up-to-date.

Your assessment of the situation needs to include an examination of the current family situation. What is happening in this family, and how can you identify this at the onset as part of your investigation? Has there been an incident of domestic violence? Are there new stresses for any of the members? Recognizing the client's reality and empathizing with his or her situation can assist in establishing a less threatening contact.

It is important to collect as much collateral information as you can about the family you intend to visit before leaving the office. Possible sources of useful information include:

Your own agency's files on the client. Such records will show you what kinds of investigations have taken place in the past. They will also identify who else was present and what your agency currently knows about each of them. Such records should identify possible concerns such as a history of alcohol or substance abuse or a history of domestic violence. Some agencies have systems in place to "flag" potentially violent clients. This information may be kept at the front of the paper files, or may be integrated into their computer data system.

Dispatch records of police and ambulance calls to the residence. Many law enforcement and ambulance agencies now have computerized dispatch systems. These systems will quickly list what kind of calls the police and ambulance have responded to at this home in the past.

Such records will tell you if violence or weapons were involved in the calls.

Police records of arrest warrants, probation orders, criminal charges, bail conditions, history of arrests, and convictions. There may be laws and protocols that limit the information your local law enforcement agency can provide to you. Nevertheless, at the very least they can tell you:

- If the persons that you are investigating have any outstanding warrants;
- If your client is bound by certain relevant bail or probation conditions; or
- If the dispatch history indicates the need for police backup when you attend the client's residence.

Workers should familiarize themselves with the local police protocols, and the best method to access this information.

Family court records. Family courts can supply information on restraining orders, divorce/separation agreements, and custody orders that may prove useful to your investigation.

Mental health records. Local mental health teams can often inform you if a client has a history of mental disorders. They can often tell you the nature of the disorder, and possibly their opinion on the potential for violence.

Immigration records. This is a resource often overlooked by social workers. If the client is not a citizen,

Immigration agencies can tell you what the client's status in the country is. If the client is in the country illegally, Immigration officers can assist you.

Neighbors. Often the complainant in a child-welfare or mental health case is a neighbor or building manager. The fact that only one neighbor has called does not mean that other neighbors have not also witnessed incidents of concern. Canvassing the neighbors is time consuming, but it can uncover a wealth of information about a residence and its occupants. Workers need to be careful about maintaining the confidentiality of their visit and not disclosing sensitive details about the families. Often you need only tell neighbors that you have concerns about the children or adults, and then ask if they have any information to provide.

The process is complicated if the complainant does not know the names of the clients involved. It may be a citizen calling about a neighbor he or she does not know. It may be a complaint about a child in a park who appears to be covered in bruises. This presents a new set of problems, as without a name, collateral checks become more difficult. It is important to work with what information is initially available and continue your assessment as more information is gathered.

Your agency may have a system in place to cross-reference addresses with client's names. Law enforcement agencies can often check on their dispatch computers for information on the nature of previous police calls to these addresses. This may not provide you with a client's name, but it may enable you to collect some safety information. An example would be a history of previous police calls to a given address for domestic disturbances, fights, or drinking parties.

Once you attend at an address, your safety assessment needs to continue as you gather more information. As you obtain names and other identification, you need to call back to your office to determine the history, if any, of the family. You can use this information to reassess your safety in the home.

Remember that when you are conducting an investigation, gathering information is the first important step. Be alert to the possibility of inaccurate information, and try to confirm its validity. Often complainants or collaterals will have their own agenda and may provide information intended to meet their needs. Examples of this are difficult child custody disputes and landlord-tenant disputes. Although complaints that are of a malicious nature still need to be investigated, be cautious in drawing conclusions. You should exercise extra caution if the complainant is anonymous.

Another important consideration is the ethnic and linguistic background of the client. Make sure that you are familiar with the customs and taboos of the ethnic group that your clients come from. A comment or gesture that is innocuous in your culture may mean something quite different in somebody else's. If there is any chance that somebody in the residence speaks a language that you do not understand, it is prudent to have an interpreter along to assist. This may not seem necessary if the client speaks your language, but in times of stress and crisis, persons often resort to their language of origin. As well, the client who seems helpful and cooperative could pass instructions to another party in a language you don't understand that may compromise your safety without you being aware of it. The authors have often encountered situations where the clients were fabricating an alibi among themselves in a foreign language while feigning a lack of English language skills. Having a colleague or interpreter with you who understands the language will reveal such deceptions. Incidents have been recorded of workers being attacked by friends or family members called to the residence by a client who made a seemingly innocent phone call in a language the workers didn't understand. Had they known what the client was up to, they could have taken steps to protect themselves.

A recent example involved a pair of workers who attended at a residence to apprehend an Asian child. This was the child's grandmother's residence. The parents that posed the risk to the child did not reside there. When the workers arrived, the grandmother presented as cooperative and friendly. She excused herself to conduct a telephone conversation in a foreign language. She did this within sight and hearing of the workers, but as they did not speak the grandmother's language, they did not realize that what she was really doing was phoning the child's father, a gang member, advising him to intervene. Just as the workers were getting into their car with the child several carloads of gang members armed with baseball bats pulled up. The workers were boxed in and the gang members smashed out the windows of their car. Fortunately the workers had a cellular phone and called 911. Police arrived and arrested these parties just as they were climbing in the windows of the worker's car. Fortunately these workers escaped without injury.

If these workers had taken an interpreter with them in the first place, they may have escaped without incident. I recall another incident in which a client was overheard by a court interpreter. The client was threatening to "wait outside and do something to that worker." The worker was able to notify the court sheriffs to deal with this situation.

Conducting adequate background checks beforehand may be time consuming, but so is filling out incident reports, insurance claims, and compensation forms following a violent incident. Which would you rather spend your time on?

Chapter Four Summary

- Never assume. There is always something about a situation that you do not know.
- If it is unsafe for a child, it is unsafe for a worker.
- Field investigations begin at your office.
- Do background checks.
- Is your information accurate and recent?

PART TWO

REDUCING THE RISKS

5. Having the Client Visit the Office

Out of this nettle, danger, we pluck this flower, safety.
—William Shakespeare

The decision whether you interview your clients at their residences or have the clients visit you at your office affects the level of risk involved. There are a number of safety concerns that make office visits an attractive alternative:

In a client's residence you have little control over distractions. The client's residence has all kinds of distractions such as televisions, radios, or children's video games. In the middle of your interview one of the client's friends or associates may phone. At the very least this is an unwelcome distraction. In a worst-case scenario this caller may counsel your client to throw you out. Associates or friends of the client could suddenly show up. They may not be as sympathetic to you as the clients and may interfere with your work or incite the clients to violence. Whether you are in a discussion or in a physical conflict, you'll have difficulty prevailing if you are outnumbered. Home visits leave you very little control over problems like this, which can seriously compromise your safety. In an interview room at your office you don't have to worry about these distractions.

You have no control over the environment that you are entering. Client's homes are often cluttered. Any number of things are within the client's reach that he or she could pick up and use as a weapon should the situation become violent. Clients may even have weapons secreted in their residence that they could suddenly produce if things look bad for them. This is another headache you can avoid in an interview room back at your office.

Distance can be a factor. The client's residence may be situated a long way from both your office and the nearest police assistance. This is especially true in rural areas.

As you can see, you will have less control over the interview process if you conduct an interview at the client's home. The potential for distractions and interruptions is high. By using an interview room at your office, you can eliminate all kinds of safety concerns and distractions.

This does not mean that an interview at your office is automatically safe. There are still concerns and things you can do in the office to make the situation safer. The room at your office in which you interview the client should be well lit and uncluttered. Earth tones for the walls are best for their soothing influence. A calendar on the wall is useful. The room should be free of anything such as metal toys or glass ashtrays that an irate client could use as projectiles. If there is a phone in the room, it should be secured to the wall or table to prevent it from being picked up and thrown. It is useful to equip the room with windows so that other workers in the office can see what is going on inside. This could be one-way glass. Another option is having a receptionist, supervisor, or other staff member monitor the activity in the room via closed circuit TV. If recording equipment is being used, it should be hidden, but the social worker conducting the interview should tell the client that they are being recorded.

Some agencies have set up rooms for receiving especially volatile clients that have a designated entrance for the clients to enter and leave. A table separates the client from the interviewer. A separate door behind the interviewer provides an emergency exit should the client behave violently. If interviewing the client in your office, situate your desk so that the client is not between you and the door.

Having a room reserved solely for interviews is preferable to using your own office for several reasons. If you must use your office to conduct interviews, you will constantly be clearing away office equipment such as staplers, hole punches, or telephones that the client may pick up and throw. You'll have to clear away any sensitive documents or files that you don't want clients to see.

Having a room other than your office in which you can conduct interviews will eliminate this problem.

If your background investigation has revealed safety concerns, be sure to notify your supervisor prior to the client's arrival so that all of the necessary preparations for the visit can be made. Sometimes clients may call in anger and tell the social worker that they are on their way to the office. If this occurs or if the client you are expecting has a propensity for violence, be sure to let the receptionists know so that they won't be taken by surprise.

Don't schedule client visits for times such as lunch hours or training days when there will be few if any staff members around who may offer assistance to you if you need it. Be sure to notify your supervisor if you are conducting an interview or assessment in the office late in the day. People are often anxious to leave at the end of the day and you don't want to find yourself in the position of being all alone with clients in the office with no one to offer assistance if you need it.

When clients arrive, take note of their emotional state and demeanor. It is better not to even start an interview or assessment in the first place if it is clear from the outset that the client is likely to get out of control.

The reception area should be visible to the administrative staff, and there should be a locked gate or door separating it from the rest of the office. There should be signs in the waiting area that indicate zero tolerance for violence. Have clients sign in at the reception desk and escort them both to and from the office where the interview or assessment is being conducted. It has been our experience that clients wandering around the office pose a greater threat to personal safety and security. Any staff member who notices strangers wandering about the office should politely question them as to their business there. Having reception issue temporary visitor identification is a good way to control unwanted guests.

You should consider using a partner to assist you in interviewing or assessing clients. One of you will be the primary interviewer, doing all of the talking. This avoids over-stimulating the client. The other should quietly make notes and observe. This backup worker will be in a better position to observe the client's body language. The presence of an extra worker can often discourage violence on the part of an angry client; there is safety in numbers. It is advantageous to utilize a backup worker who is familiar with the client. If you are the only one who has had contact with the client, this is an excellent opportunity to introduce the client to another worker who can handle the client's concerns in case of your absence from the office.

If you become aware that the tension between you and the client is escalating, it may be time to terminate your interview. You can offer to meet with the client again at a later date when emotions have cooled, if appropriate. If clients continue to escalate or threaten violence, escort them from the building. Have other staff members assist you if necessary. It is a good idea to develop a system of innocuous phrases or gestures that you can use as a signal to summon assistance without alerting the client. One signal may indicate that you require the assistance of another staff member. Another may indicate that you require the immediate assistance of the police. Such signals can be passed using your office's paging system, intercoms, or telephone. It is a good idea to have the interview room equipped with a hidden panic alarm button for cases when you are interviewing volatile clients.

In chapter four we discussed the different levels of priority assigned to calls by police dispatchers. It is essential to pass on all of the pertinent information when you call 911 in order to ensure a timely and appropriate response. A recent example of this involved a situation in which a client became violent and began to trash the waiting room inside the office. A social worker called 911 and reported that "a man has trashed the office." She didn't mention that the man was still there wrecking the place. The dispatcher didn't think to ask. Assuming that the perpetrator had left, the dispatcher entered this incident on the dispatch list as a report call. A police unit would attend as soon as they had dealt with more serious calls.

Fifteen minutes later the man was still breaking up the office and several social workers were trying to restrain him. The social worker called 911 back frantically, demanding to know why the police hadn't arrived yet. It was only then that the 911 dispatcher found out that the offender was still at the office. The police were dispatched to the office and the client restrained.

If you have to call 911, tell the operator everything that you can about the situation. If the perpetrator is still there, stay on the line. That way you can pass on updated information to the dispatcher, who can, in turn, update the attending peace officers. Give the dispatcher the name and description of the party who is the subject of concern. This will help the attending officers quickly locate this party, especially if there is a crowd of office staff surrounding the out of control client.

Ensure that all of the office doors are locked at the end of the business day. Don't prop exits open for any reason.

Interviewing clients in the office reduces the chances of violence and affords more protection for the worker. However, there are many circumstances where home visits are necessary and more convenient for the clients. The next chapter will discuss safety issues involving home visits.

Chapter Five Summary:

- It is hard to control the environment in the client's residence.
- Take into consideration the distance the client's residence is from support or assistance.
- Interviews at the office are generally safer than interviews in the field, but there are still safety concerns.
- Remove all unnecessary items from the interview room and secure everything that you can to eliminate weapons of opportunity.
- Don't schedule client interviews for lunch hours, training days, or the end of your shift: At these times there are likely to be few workers around that can assist you if you require it.
- Interview with a partner.
- Don't start the interview if the client is agitated or belligerent.
- Don't continue an interview if the situation becomes uncomfortable.
- If you have to call 911, make sure you pass along ***all*** pertinent information.

6. Attending the Client's Residence

All I'm trying to do is not join my ancestral spirits just yet.

—Joshua Nkomo

Home visits are an important part of a social worker's job. Interviews and assessments in a client's own environment will be more comfortable for the client. Families with small children, the elderly, and the infirm may have difficulty attending the office. Visiting them can reduce their stress and foster a more supportive relationship.

As well, there are a number of issues that cannot be resolved without a visit to the client's home. Often a home visit is necessary to accurately assess the client's situation first hand or to verify that the client is complying with supervision orders or care plans. We have all encountered clients who make a pretense of compliance, while continuing with whatever activities caused concerns in the first place. Another scenario is when the initial abuse or neglect complaint is made by some concerned citizen. Often the complainant does not know the names of the people they are concerned about, and neither do you. The only way to assess the situation is to go to the home in question and check it out. As we mentioned in the previous chapter, there are all kinds of safety variables inherent in a home visit over which you have little or no control. Therefore, you must adopt strategies that reduce the risks posed by these situations.

Very few of your visits to a client are likely to be surprise visits. Even so, there are many circumstances where a field worker will be arriving unannounced at a residence. You may be conducting a new investigation. The client may not have a phone. A surprise visit may be required as part of your investigation.

It is always wise to avoid rushing into a situation. Things unknown to you may have occurred before your arrival that may have radically altered the situation you expect to find. What you do before you enter a client's home can help in reducing your personal risk. Remember, it is wise to do background checks before visiting a client in order to have a better idea of what you are walking into.

One of the most dangerous parts of any home visit is your first contact with a family and their residence. You may have done your homework, including looking up the history of the client involved. You may have been in phone contact with them prior to your visit. Nevertheless, until you get inside the client's home you have no idea exactly how many people are inside, who they are, and what their state of mind is. We will look at things you can do to reduce the risks involved. The other dangerous part is when you take action that the client may not like. You should make a decision whether or not certain actions should occur during the current visit. The decision to take backup is partially based on this consideration.

Always take into consideration the history, and cultural and ethnic makeup of the neighborhood that you are visiting. Social workers should not attend communities in which there is a high rate of violence unless they have police assistance. You should consider conducting interviews and investigations in safer territory. Always be thinking about safety when approaching a situation. Plan ahead. Anticipate the opportunities a violent client may have to harm you and the ways that you might avoid or respond to this violence. If an attack comes, you won't have time to think rationally. You will fall back on instincts and planning. Next we will look at the details and some special considerations.

Residence Risk Assessment

Always have a contingency plan before you make your approach to a client's residence. Remember: If suddenly attacked, you will automatically fall back on whatever plan or contingency you have rehearsed or selected beforehand. Bob Lindsey, a well-known police trainer, once wrote,

"When you are mentally prepared, a plan allows you to instinctively react in a high stress event when there is no time to think."[100] If you have not prepared, you will be left in a very vulnerable position, wasting valuable time wondering what to do. Planning for the unexpected will leave you in a much better position to respond. Here are a few of the things that you need to consider:

- How do I approach the client's house?
- What other resources might I call upon if necessary?
- What escape route will I use if it becomes necessary to leave in a hurry?
- What cover is available to me should the need arise?
- How close is help if things go bad?
- Is the neighborhood I am visiting safe?
- Will residents in this neighborhood help or hinder me?

The first step in attending a home is to make a risk assessment. This gives you the opportunity to see how the home is situated and to develop contingencies such as escape routes. It also gives you an opportunity to get some idea of how many people are inside and what they are doing. Even if you prearranged the visit and the client is expecting your arrival, it is a prudent precaution. There is no telling what might have changed since your last contact with the client.

Anticipate the address you are looking for as you approach it. Park your car three or four doors away on the same side of the street ***before*** you reach it. **NEVER**

PARK IN FRONT OF A RESIDENCE. There are three reasons for this:

- It announces your arrival.
- It gives the evasive client an opportunity to leave by another door.
- It places you in a vulnerable position.

Also, if you need to leave the home in a hurry, it is best that your vehicle not be directly out front of the home. Keep your keys handy in a pocket so they are easily accessible.

You should leave your vehicle in a position that allows you to drive off quickly if you should need to. Don't park where you might get blocked in. If the street is a cul-de-sac or dead end, consider positioning your car so that it is facing ***away*** from the dead end. This will leave your vehicle in a better position should you need to make a quick departure. Avoid parking your vehicle in high-risk areas like alleys or in areas that may conceal suspicious people close to your vehicle.

Take a moment before getting out of your car to assess your surroundings. Keep the doors and windows locked. Look around you and listen. Do you see anyone acting suspicious? Is this neighborhood safe? Do you see people with whom you've had unpleasant experiences in the past? Is this situated close to a residence where some difficult client lives whom you may encounter on your way to your assessment or appointment? In some neighborhoods a visit by a person in authority may be less than welcome, even if that person in authority is unknown to them. If there is a lot of drug activity in the neighborhood, you may become a target for opportunists looking for money to support their addiction.

If you don't like the looks of the situation, consider driving away. Go to a safe location and request police backup. Arrange to meet the police at a safe location. Don't wait for police in an area that is unsafe. Once police arrive, they can accompany you back to the residence.

Be careful what you leave in your car. Avoid leaving documents in plain view that may announce your identity and purpose. If it is your own car, don't leave anything with your name and address in plain view. Don't leave anything in plain view that might tempt a thief. If you can, leave nothing visible in the car at all.

When you exit your vehicle, don't slam the door. If the clients are not expecting some sort of visit, this may cause them to look out of their window to investigate the noise and prepare for your visit. Quietly closing the door reduces this risk.

Study the client's residence before you approach it. Use all of your senses to evaluate it:

- What can you see?
- Can you see how many people are inside?
- Can you see or hear people fighting or arguing?
- Are there signs of violence such as broken windows or doors?

- Is there evidence of drinking, such as empty beer or liquor bottles?
- Is the entrance door closed, ajar, or open?
- Are there vehicles in the driveway?
- Can you smell drugs which may be impairing the judgment of those inside?
- Can you hear anyone in the back yard?

Don't rush in! Stop, look, and listen. Take your time and carefully observe the residence and surrounding area from a safe position for a few minutes. As you approach the client's home, you should be in the habit of automatically identifying possible escape routes that could be used in an emergency. This way you can react immediately if something goes wrong. That way, if the situation suddenly deteriorates, you will not have to take valuable time to find ways out.

If it is an apartment building, take a moment to figure out where the client's apartment is situated inside the building. If the client's apartment is situated so that it overlooks the place where you have parked your car, you may want to move it. Study the apartments around the client's apartment. Are there obvious signs of drug use/trafficking, criminal activity, or noisy parties in progress? The occupants of such apartments may act as backup to your client if your client becomes violent.

Cover, Concealment, and Escape Routes

Always have a contingency plan before you make your approach to a client's residence. As we pointed out earlier, a person who is suddenly attacked will automatically fall back on whatever plan or contingency he or she has rehearsed or selected beforehand. If you have neither selected nor rehearsed such a plan, you will be left with a basic "startle response." This is rarely an appropriate response to an attack. Planning for unexpected trouble will leave you in a much better position to respond.

In formulating such contingency plans, understanding the difference between cover and concealment is important. This is a key concept of safety training for law enforcement personnel and is equally applicable to helping professionals. Cover and concealment are two entirely different things. Concealment refers to something that will conceal you from the client. Cover refers to something capable of stopping bullets if the client appears with a firearm. Concealment is different from cover. All cover affords concealment, but not all concealment affords cover. Objects providing concealment will hide you, but not protect you.

Darkness is not a good substitute for concealment. The headlights of an unexpected automobile or an outside light fixture with a timer or motion sensor can instantly defeat nighttime shadows.

The Approach

- After you have evaluated the residence and formed appropriate contingency plans, it's time to approach the residence. Watch and listen carefully as you approach and pause at the client's door to listen some more:
- How many voices can you identify?
- What are the people inside saying?
- Does the tone and volume of their voices give you any clues about their mental state?
- Can you hear people fighting or arguing?

Use your eyes, if you can, to see inside the home to determine the number of people present, and what they are doing. A word of caution, though, avoid taking long looks through windows. It just makes you a good target.

Avoid the "ostrich effect." Just because you can't see the client does not mean that the client cannot see you. People often make this mistake around buildings with reflective glass. The client's perspective is likely to be quite different from yours. A client inside can see out of a window without standing in front of it in plain view.

Stay conscious of your surroundings. If the client became aware of your arrival, he or she may have left the residence and hidden elsewhere about the property. The client may have done this to evade you. Yet it is equally possible that clients may do this to give themselves a better vantage point for some activity that would compromise your safety. Be alert to all possible hiding places, such as garages, tool sheds, rooftops, and vehicles. As you knock at the door, don't assume that the client will open it. The client or a friend of the client may circle the house from some chore in the backyard and come up beside or behind you. Look around corners of walls and buildings before you walk around them. Always be sure of what you are walking into.

If it is an apartment building that you are visiting, you may not want to announce your arrival to the client prior to arriving at the door of the apartment. Instead of ringing the client's apartment from the entrance intercom, you might consider ringing the manager to let you in. This will give you the opportunity to listen at the client's door before knocking to get an idea what is going on inside.

The approach to an apartment doorway is similar to the approach to the door of a house. As an additional precaution, you should check the hallway outside the client's apartment. Check the hallway exit doors to see that they are not concealing a person who may be hostile. You also want to ensure that the hallway doors are unlocked in case you need to use them to escape quickly. You're not going to be waiting to take the elevator down to the ground floor if you've got some irate client after you. You don't want to encounter intoxicated people camped out on the landing or addicts using drugs in the stairways if you have to get out of the building quickly.

We remember a case that we dealt with where the police had made several visits to an apartment to investigate domestic disputes during the course of an afternoon. Twice an intoxicated male had fled from the building when police arrived. When we came on duty, we were asked by the officers involved to check this apartment where a known client with a child was residing. Everything seemed quiet when we arrived at the client's door in the hallway. But out of habit we checked the exit door only six feet away to see that the exit stairs were clear before we knocked on the client's door.

They weren't. A snarling German shepherd attacked me as I opened the door. The client's intoxicated boyfriend had positioned himself on the exit stairs with a case of beer and his dog with the intent of setting the dog on the client if she left her apartment. Fortunately this male had passed out, so he had not let the dog out when we first arrived at the client's door. I was able to slam the door on the dog and request assistance to remove both the dog and the male.

If you are approaching a residence with a backup worker, avoid moving in side by side. Spread yourselves apart a bit. Maintain eye contact with your co-worker. Communicate with your co-worker as you approach. Don't assume that your co-worker sees and hears everything that you do. If you identify an imminent threat, shout out a warning immediately.

Remember: IF IT DOESN'T SOUND OR LOOK SAFE, GET OUT! CALL FOR POLICE ASSISTANCE!

Firearms Considerations

The legal right to own firearms varies throughout North America and Britain. Some communities and cities have only a few shootings a year; others have a few every day. In many rural communities, especially those that rely on hunting as a source of income, food, or recreation, firearms will be commonplace. In a study concerning violence against health and social workers, the U.S. Occupational Safety and Health Administration found that the prevalence of handguns and other firearms is as high as 25% among patients, their families, or friends. Workers in areas where firearms are commonplace may therefore have a greater tolerance for the presence of weapons. However, as the old saying warns us, "Familiarity breeds contempt." Social workers should still insist that clients keep weapons out of sight and reach while they are present in the home. Again, checking with the local police to determine if there is a documented history of violence or weapons offenses should become routine under these circumstances.

Rural Settings

Some important safety considerations are specific to rural social work. Big problems can happen in small places. Scalera reported in 1992 that most fatal incidents involving social workers occurred in rural or suburban settings, rather than urban environments.[101] In large geographic areas, isolation and sparse populations can introduce new concerns for workers. Circumstances may often require workers to drive long distances in inclement weather. Rural offices may have low staffing and may not be able to team you up with a colleague. Emergency response units may not be nearby.

Under these circumstances, the need to have your agency aware of your location always takes on greater importance. Smaller communities often do not have house addresses. Homes are often located only by cross-streets, color of the home, and proximity to a nearest landmark. If your agency covers a large rural area, but there are smaller law enforcement posts nearby, let them know of your arrival. Tell them your purpose in their community before you visit the client.

In rural communities, two-way radio communication will probably replace cellular phones. Ensure that you have predetermined check-in times with your agency, probably more than once if you are gone for a lengthy time. Have a full tank of gas, and make sure that your vehicle is equipped with safety gear, including a spare tire, flares, blankets, water. Be sure that your vehicle is in good working order. Check the weather forecasts, and plan to stay longer than anticipated. Have a credit card in case you have to make an overnight stay.

Threats against workers in rural communities also place the worker's spouse and family at risk. The client usually knows the worker's home address and which school the worker's children attend. When anonymity in a community is not possible, and an unlisted phone number provides no protection, threats need to be treated more seriously, as clients can more easily carry them out.

Again, firearms will be commonplace in many rural communities, especially those that rely on hunting as a source of income, food, or recreation. This does not mean that workers should be accepting of their presence. Asking the client to remove them from the room or to lock them in storage is a reasonable request. Cite your own safety and comfort level. You should always make police checks when attending residences where you know there are firearms. Workers need to assess their own comfort and safety level based on the knowledge that there are weapons present. You may decide to terminate an interview, conduct it in a safer or more public place, or involve police.

In some rural areas, there is an increased growth in militant groups who are typically suspicious and hostile toward government officials.[102] They may see child protection action as unwarranted and unconstitutional government interference, thereby giving them justification for an attack on the worker.

Drug Labs

Marijuana grow operations and drug labs are increasingly common in both urban and rural areas. People operating such "grow-ops" or labs are often the target of rival operations, and thus often resort to extreme measures to protect themselves. One of the things to be looking for in your background checks before attending a residence is any history of involvement with grow operations or drug labs. Be on the look out for houses with more than the usual amount of security/surveillance equipment and alarms. Watch for possible booby traps or warning devices. Look for windows blocked off or boarded up and for excessive condensation on windows. Be suspicious if you discover rooms or whole sections of the house partitioned off or locked up. Listen for the sounds of ventilating fans and equipment. Be aware of unusual smells or vapors or the smell of mold that may indicate the presence of a drug lab or marijuana grow operation.

Such grow operations or labs are full of toxic and sometimes explosive chemicals. The best course of action if you suspect that you are entering or in such a site is to get out immediately and notify the authorities.

Dogs

Many clients own dogs as pets. Some have them to keep unwanted people away from their door. Dogs usually bite out of fear, a dog that is baring its teeth and repeatedly licking its lips is afraid of you and more likely to bite. If you encounter a dog on your approach to the client's house, use caution. Don't enter the yard unless you are certain that you can approach the house safely. If alerting clients to your arrival is not a safety issue, go to a safe place where you can call the clients by phone and ask them to restrain the dog. If the clients do not have a phone or if there is a safety issue, you may want to call for police backup at this point.

Taking the slow and cautious approach to the client's residence will often prevent you from walking into a situation that you are ill equipped to handle. Dealing with a situation is always easier if you have the opportunity to prepare for it in advance. Maintain your safety awareness throughout your contact with the client. The advantage of surprise should be yours, not the client's.

Chapter Six Summary

- Do background checks for firearms.
- Do a safety assessment of the neighborhood that you are attending.
- Make sure your vehicle is serviceable.
- Don't park in front.
- Position your vehicle to facilitate a quick departure.
- Don't leave valuables visible in the car.
- Make contingency plans beforehand.
- Identify escape routes.
- Identify safe approach routes.
- Know the difference between cover and concealment.
- Darkness is not a substitute for concealment.
- Stop, look, and listen.
- Study the residence and your surroundings carefully.
- Don't rush in.
- Identify possible indications of drug labs or marijuana grow ops.
- Don't bunch up.
- Communicate! Your co-worker may not see what you see.
- Leave immediately if the situation becomes unsafe.

7. Initial Contact and Entry

Those who in quarrels interpose,
Must often wipe a bloody nose.

—John Gay

Any police officer who deals with domestic violence will tell you that the initial contact with a client is one of the most vital and risky parts of an investigation. The same is true for social and health care workers. The first contact will affect how the entire interview unfolds.

Our first contact with our clients in the field is at their door. It is our practice to never stand in front of the door when knocking. There are a number of reasons for this. The most serious is that doors offer no protection from firearms. Standing in front of the door places you in the most likely line of fire. Of course, if you knew that someone inside was armed and dangerous, you wouldn't be standing in front of their door at all. You would have called the police and taken appropriate measures to ensure your safety. Yet you don't always know what is on the other side of that door.

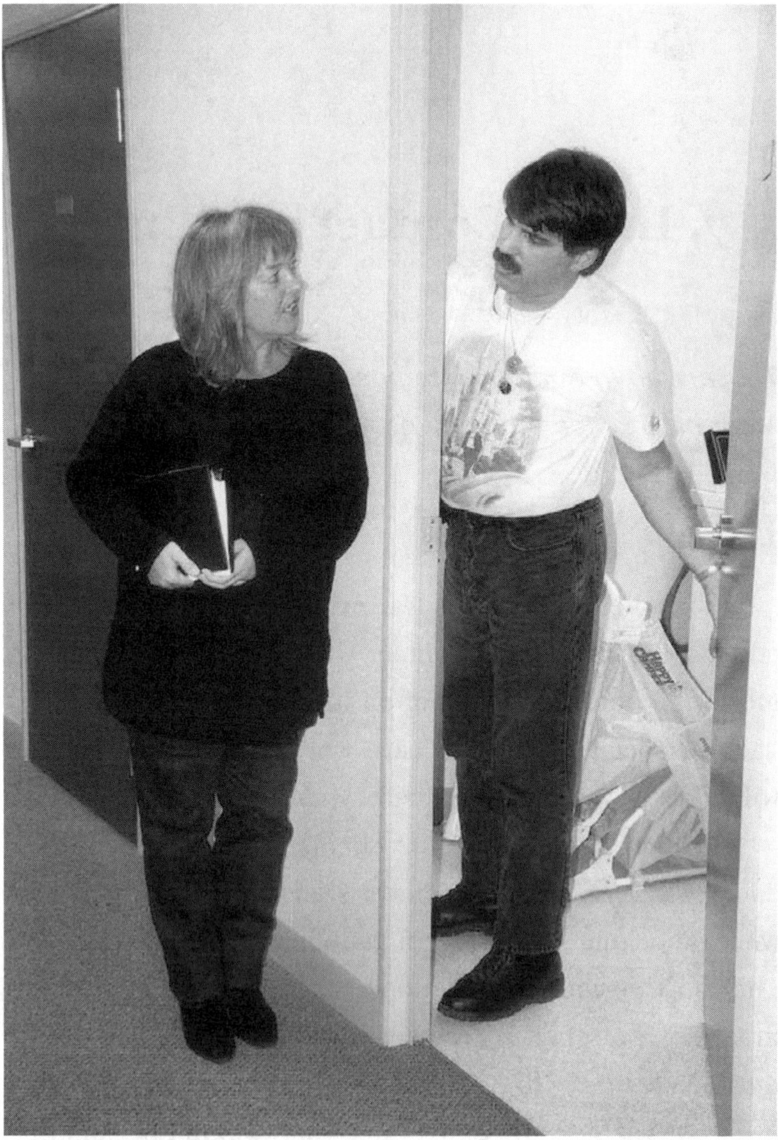

Figure 1: Standing on the hinge side of the door, forcing the client to open the door all the way.

In the last chapter we pointed out how a social worker often has to visit homes to investigate initial complaints in which the names and backgrounds of the occupants are unknown. Standing to one side of the door is a safety habit that will take care of these unknowns and uncertainties.

Another concern is that some doors open outwards. Standing in front could result in you getting knocked over when the door is opened. The other concern is the amount that you will be able to see once the client opens the door. The primary worker should stand against the wall on the doorknob side of the door. This forces the client to open the door completely to see you, and allows you to see in (Figure 1). You will be able see the room behind the client, revealing the presence of additional people and the state of the room. If what you see raises safety concerns, you can now take appropriate action. If you stand on the other (hinge) side, clients can open the door a crack and peek out, concealing the client and the inside of the house (Figure 2). You won't know what you are walking into until you have actually entered.

We recall a case where we had arrived at an apartment to check on the well-being of a woman with children who was the victim of spousal assault. The woman told us that her abusive husband was not home. However, because of the way that we had positioned ourselves, the woman had to open the door fully to see us. This allowed us to see the living room behind her.

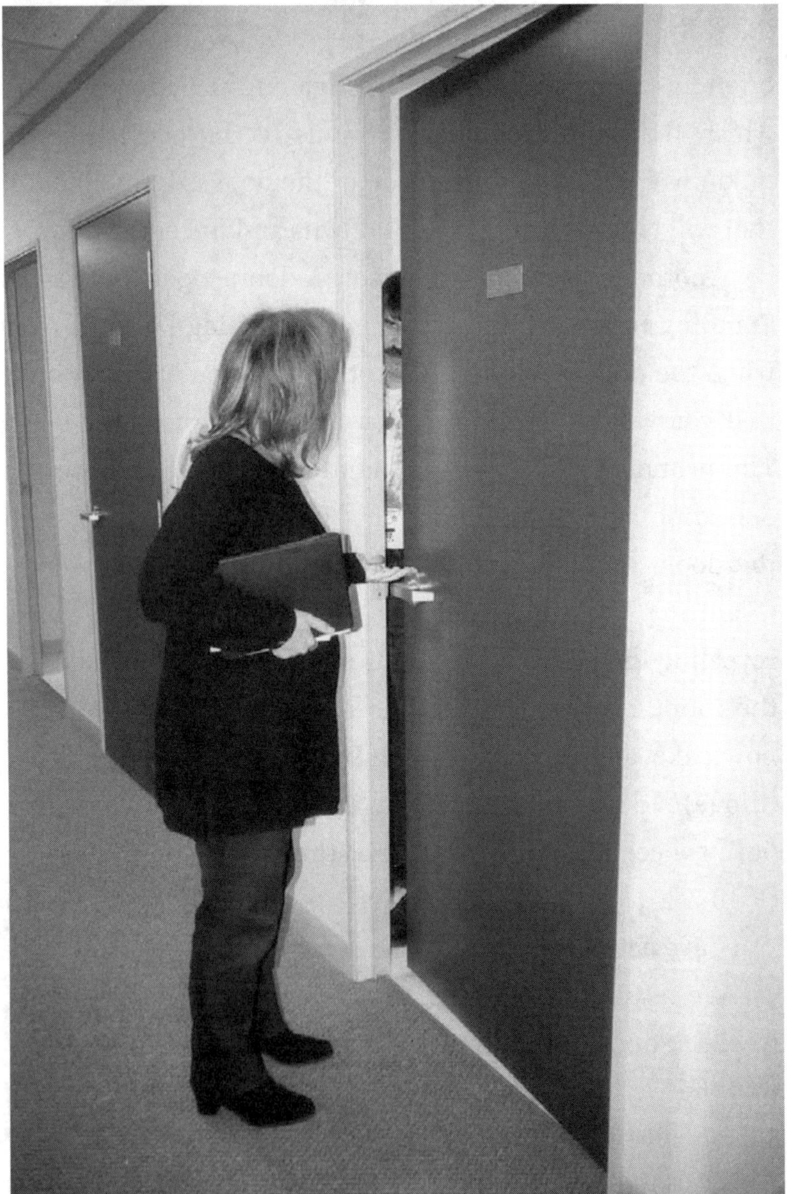

Figure 2: Standing in front of the door, allowing the client to peak out.

On a coffee table in front of the living room sofa we observed two steaming cups of coffee. Two smoking cigarettes were resting on the ashtray on this same table. We entered and found the abusive husband hiding in the hall closet. He had forced his way into the home shortly before our arrival. The victim had lied to us under duress. The husband was arrested for violating a court order prohibiting contact with the victim. If we had stood on the other side of the door, the victim might not have opened it wide enough for us to make these observations. We might have unknowingly left her in a position of extreme risk.

If you hear a dog inside the house, hold the door shut by the door handle and ask the client to secure the dog. Even if the dog is not violent, it can frequently be an unwelcome distraction when you are trying to interview the client.

Always have the client open the door. If clients ask you to come in without opening the door for you, insist that the client open it. It is best that you meet the client at the door and continue your risk assessment before you enter.

If clients say that they cannot come to the door, ask why. This is often a concern when dealing with elderly or incapacitated clients. Try to get a look inside through a window to confirm why it is that they cannot come to the door if you aren't aware of any good reason.

When the door is answered, ask to speak to the person whom you are visiting, for example, the parent. Often whoever answers the door will try to ask questions about your identity and the nature of your visit. Persons who live with the client, or are friends with them, may want to protect the client from what they perceive as "unjustified state interference."[103] Give them as little information as possible, and be non-threatening. A good approach is to introduce yourself and tell the person at the door that there are some things that you need to discuss with the client.

Once you have the clients you want to speak with at the door, again identify yourself. Give the reason for your visit and let the clients know that you would like to speak with them inside, in private. Have your identification handy so that there can be no mistake about who you are and what organization you represent. If the client is going to react negatively to your authority, this is the time to find out, not after you have entered and the door is closed behind you.

If at this point the clients tell you in a violent and hostile manner to go away, and that they do not want to speak with you, generally you should listen to them and leave. You may need to advise them that the matter is important, and that you will be returning. We have had great success at reminding people that we have a job to do, and that their refusal to cooperate does not mean that the matter will be dropped. Often once the client realizes that you mean business, and if you are being honest about your agenda, then they will often agree to speak with you.

Entry

Don't be too quick to enter the client's house. Your immediate entry could precipitate a violent reaction. Try to assess the situation inside before you attempt to enter. You can do several things to ensure your safety once the client's door is open and you are ready to enter the client's home.

1. Open the door fully, letting it bump up against the wall behind it. This ensures that no one else is hidden behind it. If the door bumps up against some obstacle, try to see through the crack between the door and frame to see who or what it is.
2. Before you enter, scan the room for people, weapons, signs of violence, alcohol or drug consumption. Assess the layout of the room. Interiors of houses are dangerous places. Lighting may be poor, cover sparse, quarters close, and obstacles numerous. You are likely to be unfamiliar with the layout. There are many blind corners and places for people to hide.
3. Assess the people inside whom you see. Do they appear intoxicated? How are they dressed? People who are dressed inappropriately for the weather or time of year are a warning sign. For example: Heroin addicts frequently wear far more clothes than the average person in hot weather as they feel cold despite the heat. Another consideration is a person wearing a jacket in warm weather to conceal a weapon in the waistband of the pants.

If you don't like what you see, ***don't go in***! Leave and request police backup. Obtaining police assistance is a better alternative than attempting to interview hostile clients alone and ending up a statistic or a hostage. The client fleeing out the back and escaping temporarily is a better alternative than an ill-conceived entry. One incident reported to us involved a worker who had requested police backup in order to follow up on a scheduled protection complaint. The worker had an extended wait because the police officers assigned to assist were diverted to another call. The worker got impatient and entered the client's home alone. The worker was flung around by the arm, verbally threatened, and intimidated by the irate client before she managed to make her escape.

If possible, don't take off your shoes. Some families insist that visitors to their homes take off their shoes at the door. You are not a casual visitor. If you are wearing them, fleeing will be easier if things get violent. If you must take them off, don't stop to collect them should you later need to get out quickly.

Once inside the home, assessing the safety of the environment again is important. Determine how many people are there, and who belongs to the family. Make sure that you know where everyone in the residence is. Ask the client if there is anyone else in the house and find out where the children are. Listen for sounds in other parts of the house. Be vigilant! Never assume that the person who answers the door is who they say they are. The suspect in a domestic assault may say he or she is a friend, relative, or babysitter to avoid prosecution.

Make sure that you know who ***everyone*** in the residence is. This is a vital part of your ongoing safety assessment. Ask for identification and make sure that the identification has not been altered. As people are identified, call back to your office to determine if there is any significant history associated with these people. The backup worker can make these calls while the primary worker continues with the investigation. This ongoing information gathering and collateral checking is not only important from a safety standpoint. It is also good social work practice. If you receive information that you are not safe, leave and get the necessary support or police backup.

Do not hesitate to request that people leave if they are not involved in the business at hand. Often they will leave with no further urging. This reduces the number of people to worry about and keep an eye on. As well, too many parties can interfere with the process. Parents may be willing to cooperate, but their friends may insist on getting involved, being hostile, and coaching the parent to refuse to cooperate. You do not want to find yourself in a situation where you are outnumbered. If you feel uncomfortable with the situation, get police backup to reduce the disparity in numbers.

It is a good idea to eliminate other distractions such as television or radios, as well. Ask the client to turn down the

TV or radio or ask permission to do it yourself. Tell them it will make it easier to attend to their concerns.

Assessment of the internal environment is an important step. Often living quarters are small and cramped, and there may be little room to move around. Do not allow any person to get between you and the exit. Leave the exit door unlocked if possible. Look for alternative exits in case someone comes in through the one you are planning to use. Try to keep clients out of arms' reach, preferably with furniture between you. Check around the room for objects that could be used as a weapon: Studies show that the weapons most often used by violent clients are the objects within the client's reach. The kitchen is often the worst room for this, so avoid conducting interviews there.

Examining the client's house may be a necessary part of your assessment. If possible, when you are alone, have the client precede you into rooms to prevent you unexpectedly meeting any unidentified persons. This also removes any possibility of accusations of theft, etc., by the client and helps you keep an eye on them. If police are assisting you, checking the various rooms in the house is their responsibility. When one of us is doing a home visit we're especially conscious of doors that are closed in the home. We tell the client we're going to check these to make sure there aren't any surprises and watch their body language and facial expression as we do so. We'll listen at each door before we open it.

Common household weapons include knives, scissors, screwdrivers, broken bottles (or bottles that can easily be broken), syringes, and pens. If you are standing in a room where there are items that could be used as weapons, remove them from the area. Do not attempt to do this without advising the clients. They may mistake your intent. Telling them that you are more comfortable putting these items away in the drawer is best. They may tell you that you are overreacting, but you will be safer. If they do not agree to this precaution, you may want to consider leaving.

If some or all of the people appear to speak a language you don't understand, try to get an interpreter to join you at the residence. As pointed out earlier, this not only reduces the chance of a misunderstanding, it will eliminate the possibility of the client passing communications that may compromise your safety without your knowledge.

On occasion you may find that an offence such as an assault has occurred prior to your arrival. You discover that the residence you have just entered is, in fact, a crime scene. If there is a suspicion that a criminal act has occurred, e.g., physical or sexual assault, involve the police from the beginning. This is because there is a strong likelihood that they can lay criminal charges, and that there are safety issues based on the allegation of violent acts.

If a criminal act has occurred, call for police assistance and, if necessary, medical assistance as soon as possible. If the suspect has left and it is safe for you to remain, try to disturb as little of the evidence at the scene as you can. If remaining is not safe, leave and go to a safe location where you can advise police and ambulance crews on what you have found.

Police Assistance

"A few parents can be dangerous to the child protection workers and others. Therefore, when a parent becomes belligerent or physically threatening, you may require police assistance to protect yourself or to maintain order. Situations of actual danger are no longer rare, and when they arise, the presence of police can prevent a tragedy."[104]

Requesting police assistance may occur at any stage of your investigation or involvement with the individual or family. Most legislation that governs social workers has clauses that require law enforcement agencies to assist social workers in carrying out their mandates or enforcing orders made by Family Courts. As well, police often assist social workers in mental health calls and hospitalizations. Many agencies have signed agreements with local law enforcement agencies outlining protocols for assistance in field investigations. There are many important factors to keep in mind when involving police:

- Clients may react negatively to the presence of uniformed police officers and feel you have overreacted to the problem.
- The increased number of persons arriving at the home can cause extra stress for the family.

- Clients may have a criminal history or outstanding warrants, and police arrival may make the focus on the social worker's assessment or investigation more difficult.

We do not intend any of the above to discourage you from calling or involving police. However, recognizing the impact that police presence may have on the clients is important. Sometimes you can achieve a compromise. For example, if plain-clothes officers are available they may be less intimidating to the client.

When coordinating a response with police, do not assume that you are clear on each other's role on the call. The officers that attend may have no experience with the procedures and legislation involved in your work. Even if they do, they may have previously worked with another field worker whose style is quite different from yours. To avoid misunderstandings, you should meet with the police before attending the home, preferably at a location out of sight of the residence. It is important to:

- Discuss the nature of the complaint you are investigating.
- Give police as much information as you have on the parties involved, such as names and birthdates. They need this to search for records in their databases.
- Advise police what you need to accomplish, and what the possible outcomes are. For example, to interview the children alone, to speak with parents separately, to

check for food or possibly to remove the children from the home.

- Discuss with police what you see their role as. Is there an allegation of a criminal act that needs to be investigated? Do you need police to speak with the parents? Do they need to do checks for criminal history? Must they search the home for weapons or drugs? You may only need police to stand by to reduce the chances of violence. In any event, they need to be clear about what your expectations are and agree on them.

Entering the client's residence is probably the most dangerous and critical stage in terms of safety. Until the door is open and you step inside, you have no idea exactly what you will find there. We must emphasize that if you do not like what you see, you should not go in. Turning away at the door is easier than getting out the door again once it has closed behind you.

Chapter Seven Summary

- Stand on the wall on the doorknob side of the door: Never stand in front of a door.
- Have the client secure dogs before you enter.
- Let the client open the door.
- Know whom you are speaking to. Deal with the client directly.
- Identify yourself.
- Don't be too quick to enter. Stop, look, listen, and evaluate.
- Scan the interior for risks before you enter.
- If you don't like what you see, don't go in.
- Leave your shoes on.
- Be sure you know where everyone is.
- Ask people who are not involved to leave.
- Limit distractions like stereos and televisions.
- Look for weapons within reach of the client.
- Involve police when it is required for safety or investigation.
- Tell the police what you are doing and what you expect of them.

8. Control

Self-defense is nature's eldest law.

—John Dryden

The space surrounding you, out to a distance of about three feet, is your comfort zone. We usually have a physical reaction when people enter our personal space; often we will attempt to back up to maintain a comfortable distance between ourselves and the person approaching. To protect yourself from physical harm you need to create an even larger safety zone around yourself that is ten to twelve feet in diameter. The more people you are dealing with, the bigger the safety zone required. Most people will avoid firearms but leave woefully inadequate distances between themselves and a client armed with an edged weapon such as a knife. The minimum reactionary gap that police officers require to draw a holstered handgun and fire upon a person who suddenly rushes them with an edged weapon like a knife is ***21 feet***. If the client grabs a stabbing or edged weapon and is within arms reach of you, chances are he will be able to stab or slash you before you have time to react.

Don't take chances. If you suspect that the client is armed, then STAY AWAY! Don't get too close. Maintain adequate distance between yourself and your client to give yourself adequate reaction time.

Clients who are upset or who want to intimidate you will often move into your personal safety zone to crowd you. If you find yourself backing away from a client, it is

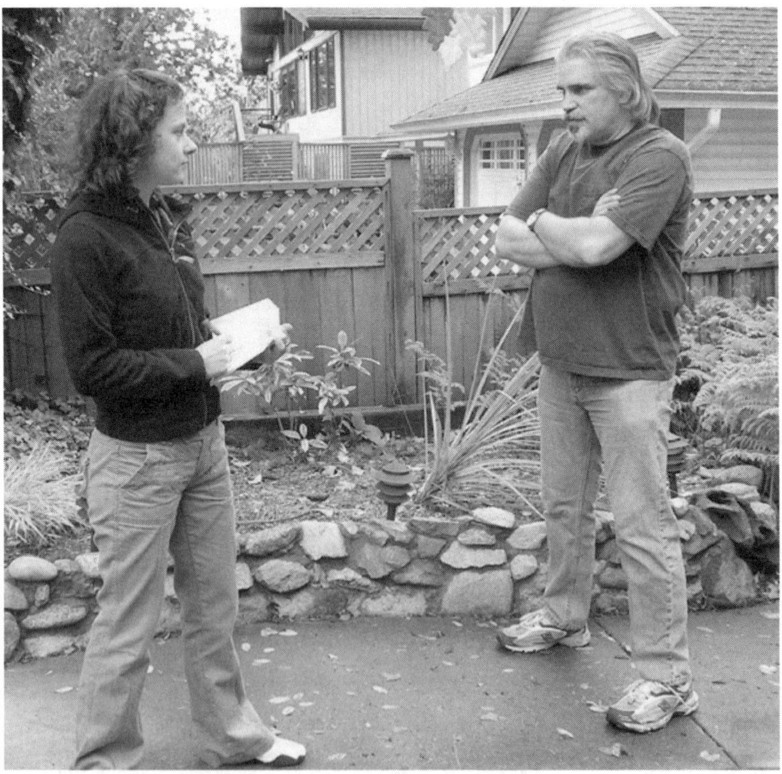

Figure 3: Interview stance with the feet at 45 degrees to the client and the strong hand in back.

important that you insist on the client staying back. If the client refuses, chances are the situation is not safe. It may be time to withdraw and request police assistance.

Don't sit in the client's house unless you are comfortable with the situation and the client is sitting, too. If the client is standing, you should be standing as well.

When standing in front of a client, adopt an interview stance to protect yourself. Stand with your feet at a forty-five-degree angle to the client, with your strong (writing hand) side farthest away, as shown in Figure 3. Position

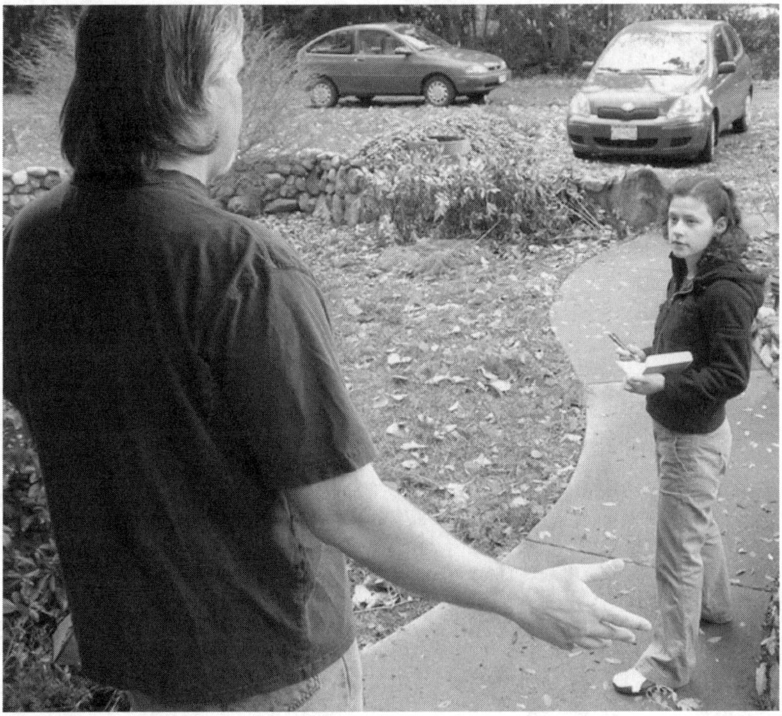

Figure 4: The interview stance makes it more difficult to attack the vulnerable parts of your body.

yourself out of the client's reach and, if possible, a little to one side. This places the most vulnerable parts of your anatomy, your face, groin, and kneecaps, in a less exposed position (Figure 4). It makes it harder for the client to strike or kick you in these areas. Using obstacles such as tables or other furniture to put a barrier between you and the client offers greater protection against attack.

Keep your hands free if possible. Keep your hands out of your pockets! You may need them to defend yourself. Don't cross your arms. The reason for this is twofold: In the first place it puts your arms in a less advantageous position should you suddenly need them to block a blow or a thrown object. Secondly, psychologically it is a "blocking" gesture that communicates the idea that you are not accepting what the client is saying. Crossing your legs communicates a similar subtle message.

Never turn your back on clients or let them go where you cannot see them. Don't let clients go off alone into kitchens, bathrooms, or bedrooms. These are the most common places to conceal weapons. For this same reason they are poor locations to conduct interviews of potentially violent clients.

Keep the client's hands in sight. Hands may be holding weapons. If you cannot see the palm of the client's hand and if the client's fingers are not all straight, the client likely has something concealed there.

Separate all parties in conflict. Tell the parties that you need them to be apart, and tell them where you want them to go. Don't touch them if you can help it, as they may misinterpret this as an aggressive act. Try to move the parties into areas where they cannot see one another. This makes it less likely that they will get into another conflict. Never stand between persons in a conflict.

If you have a co-worker with you, an option is to have all of the people in the house gather in one room. That way, your co-worker can watch them while you conduct your assessment.

If possible, always keep your co-worker in sight. Sometimes your co-worker must take a client or child into a room alone to interview them privately. Before you enter, make sure no one else is in that room. Have the backup person stay with the rest of the people present while the interview takes place.

Use a prearranged code to advise your co-worker if you see a weapon or a threat. This could be any innocuous word or phrase. Examples include: Referring to your co-worker by their surname when you usually use their given name, or telling them that you need to go to your car to get a piece of equipment. Get out as quickly as possible and call for police assistance if necessary.

The Power of the Spoken Word

Social workers entering the field usually have some education and training that focused on interviewing skills. These skills include empathy and acceptance as part of acknowledgment and feedback of the feelings of persons who are experiencing a crisis. Social workers aim to establish relationships with clients. They try to help their clients, using knowledge and skills, to work toward their goals. However, the increased requirement to meet statutory obligations has often made the ability to develop a therapeutic relationship difficult.

There is a difference between understandable and acceptable behavior and social workers need to be aware of when the client crosses the line from acceptable to unacceptable. Knowing the difference between allowing ventilation of feelings of anger, frustration, and depression vs. potentially hostile and out of control reactions which become directed toward the caseworker is critical to safe client-worker interactions.[105] Social workers need to respect the client's right to be angry, but not to be violent. It is understandable that parents will be angry when faced with having their child removed to foster care; it is not acceptable that they resort to violence toward the social worker. It is understandable that a teenage ward be upset about his lack of finances and poor job prospects; it is not acceptable that he sexually assaults his worker. It is understandable that a mentally ill person may be terrified of being taken to a hospital against his or her will; it is not acceptable that he or she stabs the worker.

Acknowledgment of a client's feelings can reduce the escalation of violence. However, workers need to be attentive to the signs of impending violence. They must know when "the line has been crossed." Workers need not be subjected to verbal abuse or sexual threats. None of this is acceptable, and should not be tolerated. It is often a sign that the situation may escalate, and is reason enough to terminate the interview and leave.

Try to use language that the client understands. Don't use a lot of technical language. Avoid patronizing or talking down to clients. Don't tell clients that they are wrong to feel the way that they do. Don't trivialize their concerns. Avoid generalizations. Try not to stand over seated clients, this is a threatening posture and may give these clients the impression that you are trying to act superior to them.

Clients can usually tell when a worker is not being forthright. Workers should be honest with clients about the reason for the visit, the nature of the allegation or complaint, and their intentions. Exceptions to this include safety issues for the worker or the client/child, and then withholding information for the short term makes better safety sense. For example, when hospitalizing a mentally ill client, it is sometimes best to wait for the ambulance to arrive before announcing your intentions.

If you notify clients of your plans before the ambulance arrives, they may become violent before there is sufficient help on the scene. Do not take any action that you anticipate will escalate the situation until you have sufficient workers and/or police present to deal with it.

If you have called police to assist you in removing a child, wait until they arrive before you notify parents of your plans. In our experience this is one of the most common mistakes made by field workers.

Take charge of the interview from the outset. Often, whoever manages to speak first gains an important psychological, and sometimes physical, advantage that they will retain throughout the encounter. Don't be afraid to tell people you are interviewing what you need to do, and what you want them to do.

When clients become verbally aggressive or threatening, workers often react by attempting to diffuse the situation, or by becoming angry and threatening them back. Some people believe that they can persuade reluctant clients to cooperate by punctuating their dialogue with threats. The idea is to appear menacing and intimidate the client into submission. This is, of course, very unprofessional conduct, but that is not the primary problem. The main trouble with verbal threats is that the client may call your bluff. The client may see through your language and see that you are really terrified and vulnerable. It is distracting. If you are getting verbose, you are probably paying more attention to what you are going to say next than to what the client may be doing. You might miss subtle clues that are vital to your safety.

Another drawback to threatening the client back is that threatening language can aggravate an already volatile situation. You might provoke a violent incident. Ideally, you should be de-escalating the situation with your words, not firing it up. You should speak forcefully, authoritatively, and sincerely in an attempt to control the situation. Be clear on your expectations, and what actions will be necessary if they do not meet them. Try not to present yourself as undecided.

Start with a low-key approach and escalate your response only if you have to. George Thompson has summarized the course of action, in order of precedence, as follows:[106]

- Ask (ethical appeal): Begin by asking for compliance.
- Set context (logical appeal): If this doesn't work, reason with them, setting the context. Show them the big picture.
- Present options (personal appeal): If necessary, present the options that the client is faced with. Don't bluff: The options must be realistic ones upon which you are prepared to act. Make sure that you don't say anything that you aren't prepared to back up. Never say something like, "This is the last time I will tell you this!" — unless you mean it! If the client calls your bluff and you do nothing, you will lose your credibility and your advantage. Being vague is better, such as telling the client that if he fails to comply, you will be forced "to take appropriate action."
- Confirm (practical appeal): If the client still won't comply, insist!
- ACT: If confirming does not work either, then it is time to act. Take whatever actions are necessary and legal to

achieve your objective safely. If that means leaving to request police assistance, do not hesitate to do it.

If the client appears to comply, do not drop your guard! Many a client has used this ploy to create an opportunity to flee with her children or to attack the worker. The authors recall an incident where a team of social workers had gone to a house to investigate child welfare concerns. The pair believed that they had convinced the parents to surrender their children to the agency for a while. The parents went about the house, apparently preparing the children to leave with the workers, who were patiently waiting in the living room. Before the workers realized what had happened, the parents had quietly slipped out the door and disappeared with the children. If they had kept an eye on these parents, they may have spotted what they were up to and taken appropriate measures to prevent it.

Be careful about the use of self-disclosure, and how many details of your personal life you reveal to the client. Examples include information about your children and spouse, possessions, income, schedules and routines, lifestyle, preferences, and beliefs. Clients who appear docile may be searching for information that they can use to target you later.

Transporting Clients

There are many different circumstances where social workers may need to transport clients, and this creates a whole new set of safety issues.

Social workers often use agency cars to transport clients. There is no telling who may have been the last person transported in the vehicle that you are using. Make a habit of searching the car thoroughly before you use it. Look under the seats and in the cracks between the upholstered seat cushions. On more than one occasion the authors have found knives, syringes, and other dangerous items concealed in these places by persons transported by workers from the previous shift. After every transport, search your vehicle again. This also ensures that the client hasn't dropped something like identification or money that you'll need to return to them later.

Social workers should never transport clients that need to be hospitalized. An ambulance or paramedic crew is better equipped to deal with medical emergencies that may occur en route. They also equip such units with restraints in case a mentally disordered or drugged client becomes aggressive.

When transporting children, their age and history are the most important factors. A small child in a car seat poses much less risk to the worker than a teen with a history of violence. You should always restrain children in seatbelts, and you should lock the doors. If you have any concerns that a small child will try to undo the seatbelt and exit your vehicle, there should always be another worker present in the vehicle.

Before getting into the vehicle with a youth who has a history of violence, have the teen or older child empty all pockets, purses, or bags. As well, pants legs need to be lifted up to ensure that no weapons are being hidden in socks or boot tops. If the police are with you, do not do this yourself. If you are not trained in how to do proper searches, you could end up hurting yourself. Any police officer will tell you that searches are one of the more hazardous things that they do, since a search brings you within the client's reach. If the client has a history of violence, this could be a concern. Even if the client isn't predisposed to aggressive action, pockets can hold all sorts of sharp objects like syringes or knives that could end up stuck in your hand. If you have any doubt about whether a person that you are transporting is armed or not, call for police backup and have the police conduct a proper search.

Seat the client or child in the back seat, behind the front passenger seat. If another worker is riding with you, the worker should sit in the back as well, behind the driver. This prevents the client or youth from easily reaching from behind and grabbing at the driver or the steering wheel.

Departure

When you return to your vehicle following a visit to a client, always have your keys ready in your hand. Closely examine your vehicle as you approach it. Look underneath, in the back seat, and on the floorboards. Has anyone tampered with it? Is someone who could harm you concealed in or around the vehicle?

Part of your contingency planning should include a plan to deal with people who may try to follow your vehicle. If you have any concerns about this, having police attend is wise. They can remain a few moments at the residence after you leave to ensure that no one follows you. They can also escort you if you have concerns about being followed.

It is a good idea to call your office or other destination and tell them when you are leaving. Tell them your estimated time of arrival and expected route so that they can make inquiries if you do not show up on time.

Being Followed. If you believe someone is following you, keep your doors and windows locked. Immediately call for police assistance if you have a cellular phone or radio. Pass on the vehicle license number, description, and the number of persons visible in the suspect vehicle. Stay on well-lighted and well-traveled roadways. Avoid stopping. Head for a place such as a police station or public building where security personnel can assist you. Flash your headlights and honk your horn to attract attention if necessary.

Summary

This is the part of the process that is closest to the original mandate of the social worker: Safe interaction with the client through psychology and verbal skills. With proper attention to detail, use of effective techniques (and a little luck) the skilled worker ***can*** keep control of a volatile situation and emerge unscathed. Yet there are some things that the field worker has absolutely no control over, luck being one of them. If your luck does run out, the ideas in the next chapter will help keep you safe.

Chapter Eight Summary

- Don't let anyone inside your comfort zone.
- Establish an appropriate safety zone around yourself.
- Use an interview stance to protect yourself.
- Keep your hands free.
- Never turn your back on a client or let them go where you cannot see them.
- Watch the hands.
- Separate all parties in conflict.
- Keep your co-workers in sight if possible.
- Tell your partner if you see a weapon or threat: Don't assume they see it.
- Know when the client has "crossed the line."
- Use clear language.
- Be forthright: Don't bluff.
- Take charge of the interview.
- Start low key and escalate your response as required.
- Know when to act and act decisively.
- Always search your vehicle before and after you use it.
- Never transport violent or medically unstable people.
- When you leave the client's residence, examine your vehicle before you get in.
- Be aware of possible pursuit.
- Don't get out of your car unless you are sure that it is safe.

PART THREE

SURVIVING VIOLENT ENCOUNTERS

9. Getting Out Safely

To survive it is often necessary to fight and to fight you have to dirty yourself.

—George Orwell

Sometimes, despite all your efforts and precautions, the situation will deteriorate. Words fail and you are left with a personal safety decision. Do you disengage or take control? There are several situations in which you must immediately make a decision and take appropriate action to preserve, first, your safety and, second, the safety of those under your protection:[107]

- **When others around you are in imminent jeopardy**. If the clients are acting out violently towards their children or members of their family, you need to take immediate action.
- **Whenever your personal safety zone is violated**. If the client is repeatedly encroaching upon your personal safety zone or is exhibiting pre-assaultive behavior (see chapter two), it is time to take action to protect yourself.

- **When the client will not voluntarily comply AND you have exhausted all verbal options.** In this case you need to stop talking and take action.
- **Whenever a matter of higher priority requires your immediate attention or presence**. For example, if the client is cooperating but another individual in the home suddenly tries to remove a child at risk, it is time to change your focus and take action.

Escape Plans and Routes

Unlike police officers, the primary responsibility of a social worker is not the management of violence. Social workers are often ill equipped and ill-trained to deal with violent situations. If things become unsafe for you **get out**! If you must leave vulnerable children or adults inside to maintain your own safety, THAT'S OK! **It is not your responsibility to manage violence.** Use the police for that function. You do have a right to defend yourself, but putting yourself in a position where self-defense isn't necessary is always better. If things get out of control, your best option is to leave. You can do several things that will speed this up:

- **Don't let anyone get between you and the exit.** Always be aware of where the possible exits are.
- **Stay as calm as you can**. Panic works against you.

If clients become aggressive, it is possible that they will storm out of the residence rather than attack you. Do not attempt to follow them; they could turn on you at any time.

Such an action by the client may indicate that he is going to get a weapon or reinforcements. It may be time to get out and call for police backup.

Escape

This is not as easy a thing to accomplish as it may appear. If a client suddenly assaults you, the shock may immobilize you temporarily. By the time you have recovered, the best opportunities for flight may have passed. Again, this is why developing contingency plans beforehand is important so that you can quickly put them into effect if needed. In the middle of a conflict you won't have time to think of such things.

There are several safety considerations if your plan is to leave. First, don't back up while in front of an aggressor. You cannot back up faster than a person can walk forward. You will be off balance and will not be able to see where you are going either. On the other hand, turning your back on the aggressor to flee gives the attacker the advantage. Not only can you not see the attacker, but the act of your turning and preparing to flee also gives the aggressor time to start forward toward you. In other words the aggressor will be in motion before you are.

If possible, you first want to get out from a position of being in front of the aggressor. Try to put something between you. Use loud verbal commands such as "stop," "get back," etc., and then begin your exit sideways or at an angle. This allows you to keep an eye on the aggressor while having a view of your escape route in your peripheral vision. You'll be able to avoid obstacles more easily. Once you are out the door, turn and run.

When you are fleeing from the residence, you may want to attract attention to your situation by yelling for help. Concerned neighbors may be able to call assistance for you. At the very least they can act as witnesses in any later legal proceedings arising out of the incident. This is not as good an option as having a backup worker with you that can summon assistance by cellular phone or radio. Nevertheless, if you are alone, it may be the only option that you've got.

In some neighborhoods yelling for help may not attract much of a response. We have seen safety policies that suggested that a fleeing worker yell "fire!" instead of "help!" While this may attract people's attention quickly, it can easily backfire. False alarms of fire are an offence in most jurisdictions. If such a false alarm precipitates a panic that results in someone getting injured, it may do more harm than good. People are more likely to be rescuing themselves from the perceived threat of fire than checking first to see if the alarm is valid or not.

Many agencies recommend carrying a whistle or other noisemaker to attract attention. The advantage of such a device is that it is likely to be much louder than the average person's voice. The sound carries a long distance. The drawback is that those hearing it may not recognize the sound as a call for help. They may mistake it for children playing or juveniles partying.

If you have succeeded in escaping from a violent encounter and have managed to elude your attacker, you may not want to make noise that will attract your attacker's attention and help the attacker to locate you again. Once you return to your vehicle you should either be calling for assistance by cellular phone or radio or driving to the nearest safe location where you can do so.

If you must retreat from a client's residence, your priority is to get out of the "danger zone," the area in which you are at risk from your attacker. When trying to get out of the danger zone, the best movements are those that:

- Confuse or immobilize your attacker,
- Get you out of harm's way quickly, and
- Take you to a safe place where you can call for assistance.

When inexperienced people hear shots, they tend to stop to try to figure out where the shots are coming from. If you hear shots, KEEP MOVING! Get out of the danger zone by the quickest and safest possible route. This is a far more important priority than knowing exactly where the shots are coming from.

Fighting Back

Fighting back is a last resort for social workers. The law allows you to use as much force as is necessary to protect yourself. However, the reality is that most workers didn't sign up with the intention of ever using violence. Social workers normally have a strong commitment to helping others, which doesn't include physical confrontations.

You must make every effort to avoid getting yourself into such a situation. Nevertheless, if a client attacks you despite your best efforts, you may find yourself in a situation where you have no choice but to fight to create an opportunity for you to break free and escape.

The decision to fight or not during an attack is a very personal one, especially when faced with sexual assault. There is no right decision; as the victim you will decide what needs to be done to ensure your survival. The important thing to remember is that the assault is NOT your fault.

While we show some self-defense techniques in Appendix B, we want to make it clear that simply reading this book will not make you a competent martial artist. You may be able to handle some situations by practicing what we show there. However, if you have concerns about your abilities in this area, we recommend studying the martial arts with a reputable instructor.

Effective self-protection training requires that the student develop learned responses through repetitious practice. There is no substitute for this, although recent studies have shown that visualization can be as effective as physical training for acquiring certain self-defense skills.

Becoming competent in such disciplines will improve your self-confidence, and the clients that you deal with will notice this. Self-confidence alone can be a powerful deterrent. Aggressive clients are far less likely to attack a person that they do not believe they can overcome easily. We must caution you however that small amounts of training with no follow up or practice can lead to a false sense of security. This is far worse than no training at all.

If you really have to fight, don't hold back. Go for it! It is your life and safety that are at stake. When the client chooses to attack, he or she has made the choice to use violence, not you. Don't worry about harming your attacker. Do what you have to and get away. Decide that you're going to survive the encounter. Once you succeed in disabling and/or breaking away from your assailant, get away as fast as you can. Don't stop to look back.

As we pointed out earlier in this chapter, an untrained person may respond to aggression by backing up. This is an even less desirable option if the client attacks you. Not only is it slow and awkward, but it keeps you in front of the aggressor. If a person lunges at you, move sideways to get out of the line of attack. Once individuals initiate an act of aggression, they will usually complete that act. Their momentum will carry them past before they can react. This gives you time and space to initiate a plan of escape.

If an aggressor is striking at you, your priority is getting out of the way. Block the blows with your arms or legs. Look around you for objects that could be used to block an attack. Examples are chairs, large books or trays, and fire extinguishers. The aggressor isn't the only person who has the option of using what is available nearby.

Police defense tactics trainer Phil Messina of Modern Warrior Inc. has an acronym that sums up the primary tactics for controlling a violent assailant: "V, W, L" (Vision, Wind, Limbs).[108] To attack you, a person needs to be in control of these three things.

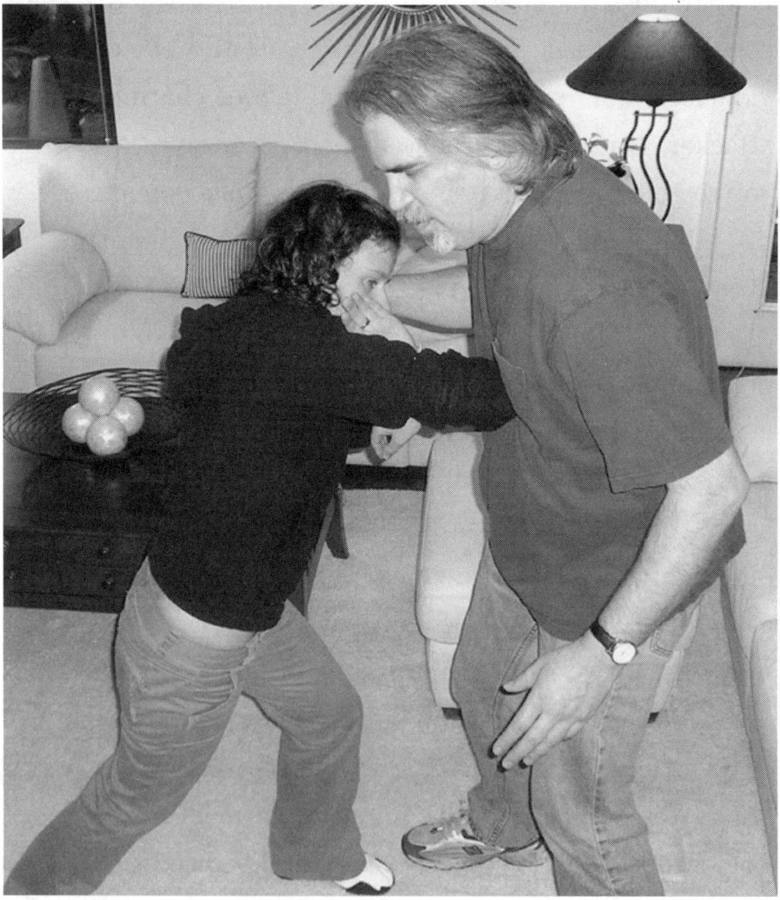

Figure 5: Reducing the attacker's wind.

A blow to the assailant's solar plexus will make it difficult for him to breathe and thus difficult to continue the assault (Figure 5). Striking or stamping on the assailant's knees or feet could put them out of commission (Figure 6). If the attacker can't stand, he can't fight or pursue.

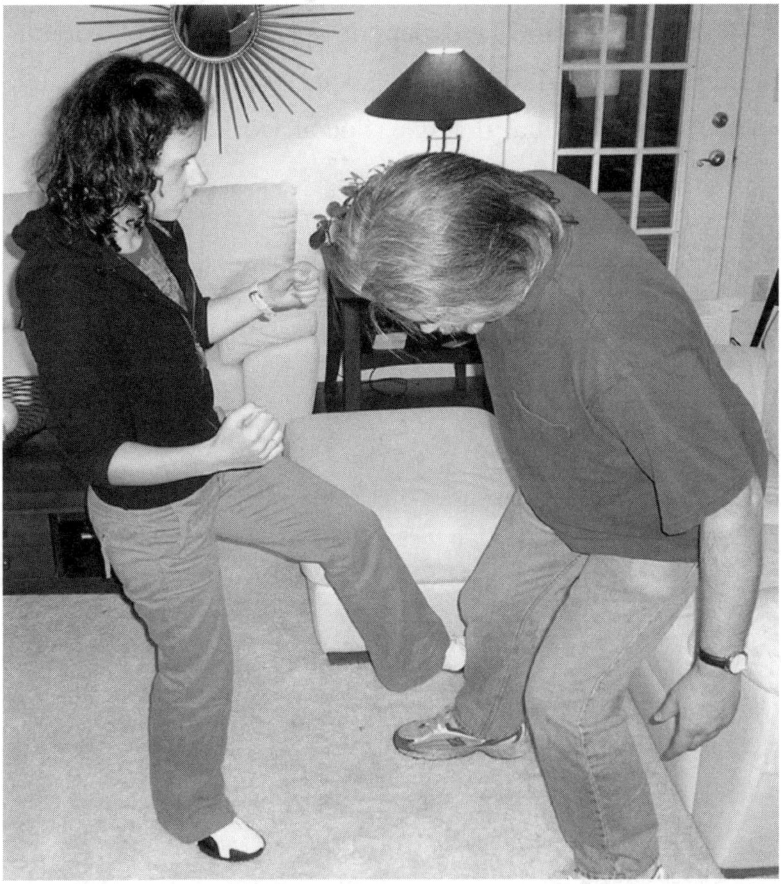

Figure 6: Interfering with the attacker's mobility by striking the limbs.

Attacking the assailant's vision is one of the most effective techniques. Even extremely violent attackers who are mentally disordered or who have high thresholds of pain can't attack you if you take away their vision. Throwing your clipboard or the contents of an ashtray in their face can accomplish this. Striking the eyes with the fingers, as shown in Figure 7, is also effective.

Earlier we mentioned pepper spray (OC — Oleoresin capsicum) and Mace. Some social workers carry such aerosols for personal defense. Social workers who choose

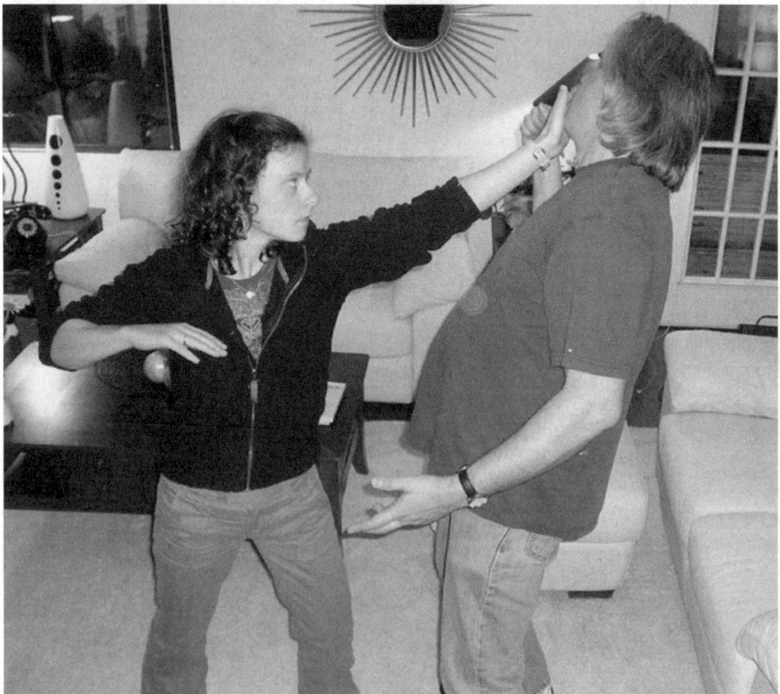

Figure 7: Interfering with the attacker's vision.

aerosol sprays as a force option for self-defense have to take into consideration several important factors. The first concern involves the way in which such aerosol agents work: You spray it in the assailant's eyes, causing pain that is hopefully sufficient to temporarily disable them. The first problem is over-spray. Some aerosol liquid may miss the assailant and hit an innocent bystander such as your partner or splash back onto you. A certain amount of airborne agent will probably get back to you if your target is upwind of you. In an enclosed space this can cause almost as many problems for the sprayer as the attacker. You aren't going to find it easy to escape from the residence if your vision and respiration are impaired.

Using a force option such as pepper spray has another drawback: It takes time to retrieve it from the purse or holder in which it is stored in order to use it. If the client suddenly attacks, you may not have time to get it out before the attacker is on top of you. If you are busy trying to fish your OC spray can out of your purse, you are probably missing an opportunity to escape. Police officers usually go into a potentially violent situation with force options such as pepper spray in their hand. Obviously this is undesirable for a social worker.

A more serious problem is that there are three categories of people whose threat will not be neutralized by aerosols:

1) Drug Addicts. People who abuse narcotics such as cocaine or morphine have a very high tolerance for pain since the substance they are abusing is a painkiller. Pepper spray may not affect such individuals.

2) Goal Oriented People: A person who is determined enough can ignore the pain induced by chemical substances such as OC, Mace, or tear gas and keep on functioning. To the average citizen, being sprayed with an agent like pepper spray is quite painful and even terrifying. This is because they have no experience with it. This explains its popularity for dealing with muggers and other members of the criminal element. However, if the aggressive client that you are dealing with is a former member of the military, chemical agents may have a negligible effect. Desensitization is likely to be one of the results of his or her training. Even an untrained individual, if he or she is enraged or determined enough, can overcome the effects of chemical agents and keep on functioning.

3) Mentally Disordered People: Like the previous categories, some mentally disordered people have a very high tolerance for pain and/or are extremely goal-oriented. Pepper spray and similar agents will have limited effect on such people.

Keep in mind point (2), above. If you are the victim of an attack by a person armed with pepper spray or Mace, you ***can*** overcome it. Your survival becomes a direct result of your determination to carry on no matter what happens. It hurts, but it causes no permanent damage and can be washed out of your eyes with saline solution or plain water later. Chances are the aerosol vapor in the air will also be affecting the assailant. Don't rub your eyes: This simply distributes the agent and rubs it in more deeply. Blink rapidly to promote tearing and carry on.

This is an unpleasant subject, but one that must be taken into consideration. Hopefully you will never need to apply the strategies discussed in this chapter if you have diligently applied the strategies discussed earlier in this book. Again, in situations such as these, the only viable option is survival. There are no rules. Losing is not an option. Do what you have to do.

Chapter Nine Summary

- Don't let anyone get between you and the exit.
- Stay calm.
- Don't pursue fleeing clients.
- Don't back up or turn your back on a client; move sideways.
- Use whistles or other noisemakers to attract attention.
- Get out of the danger zone.
- Don't get boxed in.
- If you must fight, make a decision to survive and GO FOR IT.
- Remember: V, W, L (Vision, Wind, Limbs).

10. Debriefing and Dealing with Stress

Nobody is stronger, nobody is weaker than someone who came back. There is nothing you can do to such a person because whatever you could do is less than what has already been done to him. We have already paid the price.

—Elie Wiesel

Surviving an assault creates a set of psychological problems for the worker that may last for years, long after recovery from the physical injury. The potential for emotional trauma is, in many ways, as significant as the consideration of physical injury. Many workers choose to interrupt or abandon careers in social work following an assaultive experience.[109] Rey, in 1996, noted that workers reported fear, fatigue, demoralization, sleep problems, lowered attention span, anxiety, somatic complaints, and burnout after being a target of a threat or other act of violence.[110] Most agencies that we contacted throughout

North America had some form of Employee Assistance Program or Worker's Compensation Board that was equipped to deal with the post-traumatic stress symptoms that worker's experience.

Critical incident debriefing is a crucial and necessary first step for workers after an incident of violence. The consensus in the field is that this works most effectively in reducing long-term symptoms if the debriefing can occur within 24 hours of the incident. If your agency does not provide this service, there are a number of organizations that can do this on a contract basis in an emergency.

The important thing to note here is that you must report the incident immediately, and that the management of your organization must recognize and respond to the needs of the workers. This may include providing counseling, time off from work, assistance to other workers on the team, assistance with medical costs, and referrals for legal assistance if charges are going to be laid.

The psychological aftereffects of a violent encounter can be as damaging as the encounter itself. Some of these effects are immediately apparent: crying, vomiting, incontinence, violent tremors. Most often, however, the effects are not felt until well after the incident occurs. Weeks, months, or even years later you relive and react to the incident, reviewing your actions and wondering if you were right.

The psychological strain is always greater after a violent confrontation. In the midst of an assault you will probably not be consciously aware of the stress that you are under. But afterward, when the urgency of the situation wears off, you are almost certainly going to feel some form of psychological impact.

The effects can be magnified if the assault injured you. You may end up assigned to "light duties" and reduced working hours that put a financial strain on you and your family. Your injury may make it impossible to do things around the home, forcing you to hire help and further straining your finances. Your injury may limit your ability to involve yourself in activities with your spouse and children. Your spouse, upset by the incident, may be pressuring you to switch to some safer career.

Careers in the helping professions bring you into situations in which you have to confront the worst side of human nature. This brings to an end many childhood fantasies more quickly and intensely than is the case for people in less challenging forms of employment. You may have had hopes that you could finish your career successfully without getting involved in a violent incident. Even if you were fully justified in defending yourself, you may feel that what you did was somehow "wrong" or "bad." You are likely to experience depression and a loss of innocence.

Co-workers may question your judgment or may be too busy congratulating you to notice your feelings about the matter. Supervisory personnel within your agency may be unapproachable and/or more concerned with procedures and bureaucracy than with your personal crisis. Friends in the world outside may have mixed feelings. Members of the public that you have never met, who have no appreciation of the circumstances of the incident, may write letters to the editor condemning what you did.

In the end you may feel that you are all alone. No one knows exactly how he or she will react following a violent encounter. What is known is that if you deny and repress the emotions that you are feeling following a violent incident, the effects can cause serious psychological (and sometimes physical) repercussions. From the outset you should sit down and:

1. acknowledge that a serious event in your life has occurred,
2. honestly examine your feelings about it,
3. confront what is happening, and
4. decide what to do about it.

After the incident you should be aware of the possibility of post-traumatic stress reactions. (The most common are shown in Table 1.) They may show up at any time. Sometimes they occur soon after the incident, but they may flare up when you are in another stressful situation, especially if it is somehow related to the initial traumatic event.

Some workers vow that although they were forced to use physical force to protect themselves this time, they are never going to do so again. Such an attitude is dangerous. Such a person may in the future try to calm a situation with

Table 1: Normal Post Traumatic Stress Reactions[111]

1) Sleep pattern disturbances
2) Flashbacks of the incident.
3) Development of emotional isolation.
4) Episodes of depression.
5) Fears, anxiety, and self-doubt.
6) Alienation, cynicism, and distrust.

words when a more appropriate response would be retreat or self-defense, thus landing in a worse situation than the initial assault. Making yourself a victim won't improve anything. This verges on suicidal behavior.

Nevertheless, you can prepare yourself before the event by spending some time seriously considering your job and its responsibilities. You may never need to face a violent encounter, but if the possibility is there, it should be faced.

Watch for these reactions and take positive steps to deal with them whenever they occur. Your well-being can be improved. The first person that you need to take care of in this business is yourself.

Chapter Ten Summary

- Immediately report all incidents of violence against you.
- Participate in a critical incident debriefing following significant incidents of violence.
- Be conscious of the symptoms and effects of post-traumatic stress

Conclusion

Violence against workers in the helping professions is a growing problem that will not go away. Safety awareness, preparation, and continual reassessment of situations that you find yourself in will enhance your safety. This will also reduce the likelihood of assault. Eventually it will better the profession.

Recognizing that safety is an important concern is the first important step. Workers cannot identify unsafe conditions or assess risk to themselves and other workers if their agency has not trained them in what to look for and how to work safely.[112] Workers and management alike need to focus their attention on prevention, reporting of violent incidents, and support for the workers involved. Violence should not hamper the commitment of workers to helping individuals, families, and children in crisis. Yet this reality causes persons to leave the field or it causes them to decide not to enter the field in the first place. Workers are entitled to a safe working environment, but ultimately the final responsibility for maintaining a safe environment rests with the individual.

It is our hope that this book will give you increased safety awareness and the skills needed to assess and handle unsafe situations. Worker trauma and stress are major contributors to worker "burnout" and disability leave. Reporting of violent incidents is crucial to ensuring that organizations recognize safety problems and provide appropriate support to workers to reduce the risk. With appropriate training and support, workers in the helping professions can continue to provide the high level of service that our society needs.

Safely.

Appendix A: Safety Assessment Checklist

Collaterals:

- ☐ agency files
- ☐ police
- ☐ immigration
- ☐ mental health
- ☐ complainant
- ☐ neighbors

Does your information indicate:

- ☐ a history of violence or physical abuse?
- ☐ a family member with a mental illness?
- ☐ drug or alcohol use by family members?
- ☐ that firearms or weapons may be present in the home?
- ☐ criminal activity?
- ☐ physically aggressive adolescents?
- ☐ previous complaints or investigations?
- ☐ that statutory action may be necessary?
- ☐ history of threats or aggression toward workers?
- ☐ vicious dogs or other dangerous animals?

☐ that the client speaks a different language than your own?

Equipment:

☐ a cellular phone or two-way radio, and spare, charged batteries

☐ appropriate clothing, and as few extras as possible

☐ a full tank of gas and emergency equipment in the vehicle

☐ phone numbers if 911 not available

☐ body armor if required

Prior to leaving:

☐ determine the minimum that you need to accomplish during the investigation, and what your anticipated agenda is

☐ leave the address you are attending with your supervisor, colleague, or administration staff

☐ arrange for a coworker or supervisor to monitor prearranged check-in times

☐ arrange for a colleague to attend with you, advise them of the nature of the call, and agree on safety signals

☐ carry with you only what is necessary, and what can fit into your pockets or briefcase

☐ search vehicle for contraband or weapons in case transport is necessary

Arrival:

- ☐ park your car a few doors away (not in front) in a place where you can drive away easily
- ☐ assess the residence from the outside for signs of violence, broken glass, evidence of liquor bottles
- ☐ listen for any noises from inside that would indicate a fight or violence in progress
- ☐ note possible areas for concealment and/or cover, and possible escape routes
- ☐ have your car keys handy
- ☐ have a rehearsed safety plan

Entry:

- ☐ observe if your reception indicates that the situation may escalate
- ☐ visually check the home for anything that could be used as a weapon
- ☐ know who is in the home and where they are
- ☐ maintain access to an exit

Interview:

- ☐ use your social work de-escalating skills to enable you to maintain control of the interview
- ☐ note any of your physical reactions that may indicate that you feel unsafe
- ☐ pay attention to the client's level of cooperation and the progress of the interview

- ☐ watch for any threats or physical gestures made toward you

Getting Out Safely:

- ☐ leave by the nearest exit when your assessment indicates that you are no longer safe
- ☐ abandon personal belongings if retrieving them will compromise your safety
- ☐ do not attempt to manage violence unless the client assaults you
- ☐ call for police if you have been forced to leave people in the home who may still be unsafe

Follow up:

- ☐ report any violent incident to your supervisor
- ☐ ensure that you fully document the incident in your agency's files for future reference
- ☐ debrief and get support as necessary

Appendix B: Escape Techniques

The following techniques may be used in situations where a violent client has grabbed hold of you. The contingencies illustrated include one and two-handed wrist grabs, one and two-handed lapel grabs, choke holds, bear hugs, headlocks, and hair grabs. To be competent with these techniques you should constantly practice them with your colleagues.

These techniques may not disable your attacker, but they will help you get yourself free so your options to fight or flee are enhanced. Reacting quickly is essential. It is much easier to escape if you act before your assailant has a firm grasp.

#1: One-handed wrist grab

This technique can be used to disengage yourself from an assailant who grabs one of your wrists.

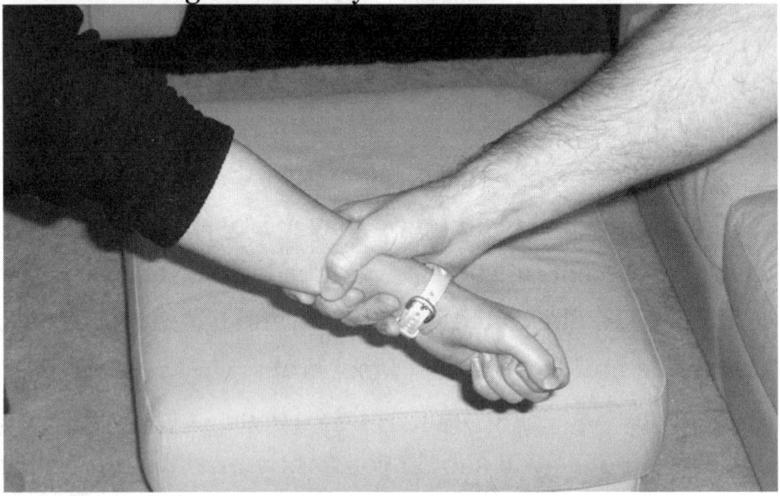

First, with your free hand, grab the hand of the arm being held...

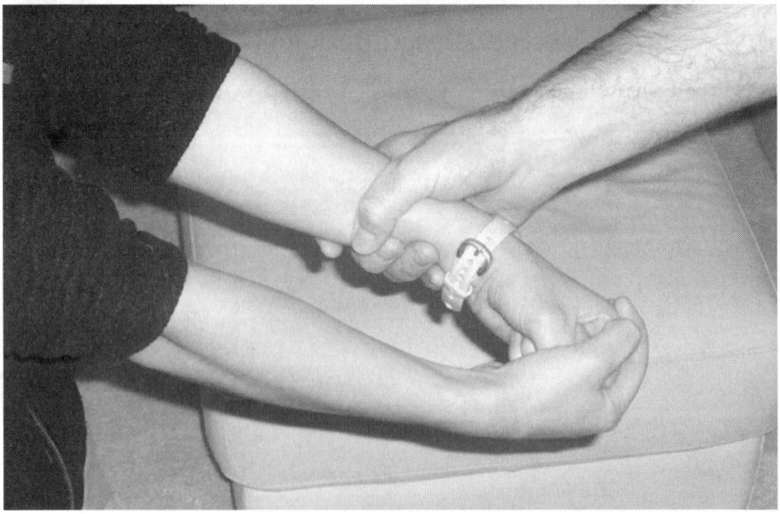

Then, using this free hand, pull the arm being held towards you, levering the arm against the assailant's thumb, which is the weakest part of the assailant's grip...

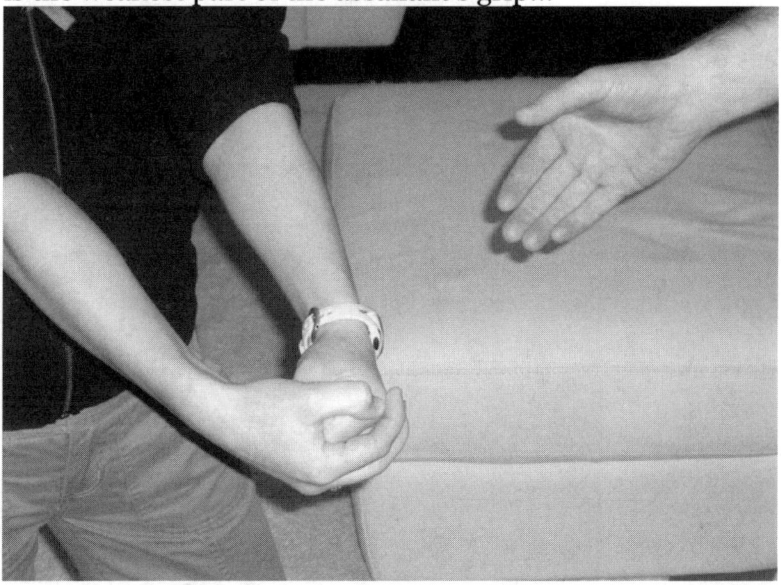

This should pull your arm free of the assailant's grasp.

#2: Two-handed wrist grab

This technique can be used to disengage yourself from an assailant who grabs your arm with both hands.

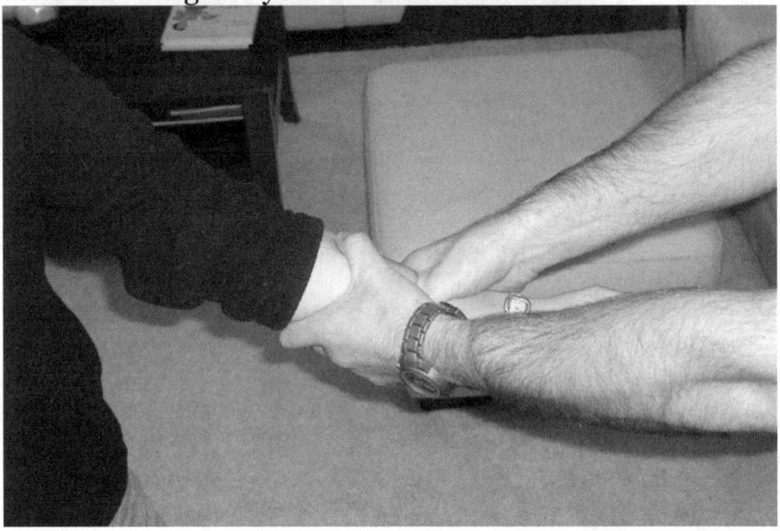

First, with your free hand, reach between the assailant's arms and grab your other hand...

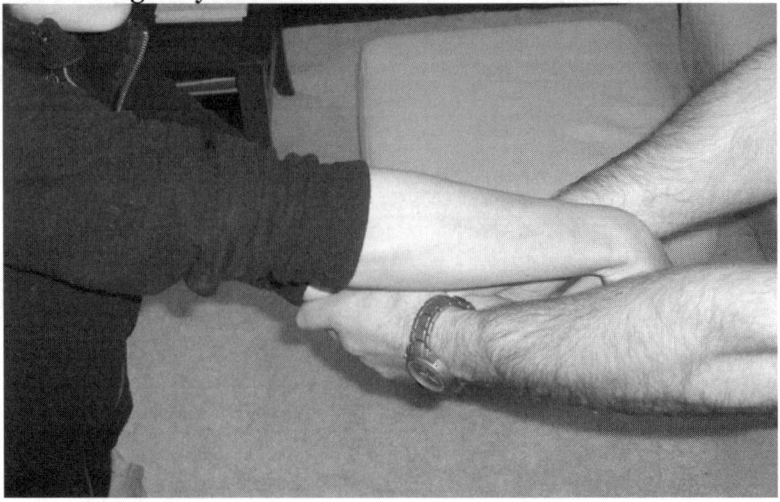

Then, simultaneously pull towards you with your free hand and bend the arm being held at the elbow,

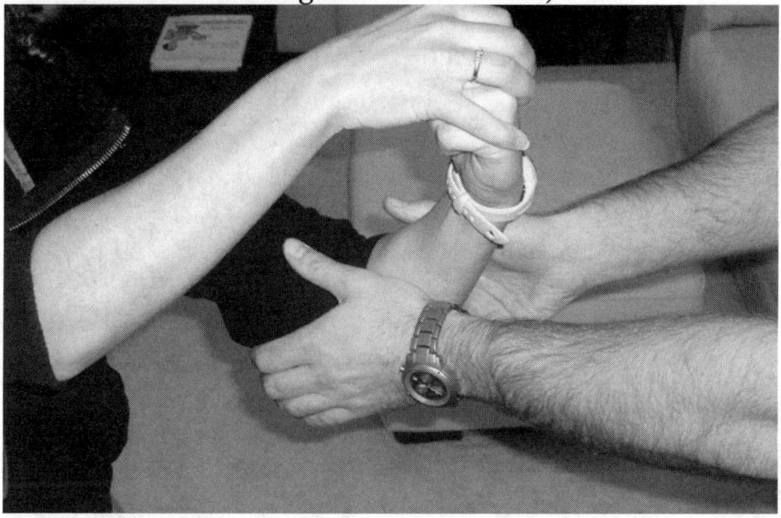

bringing this elbow up sharply into the assailant's sternum or chin...

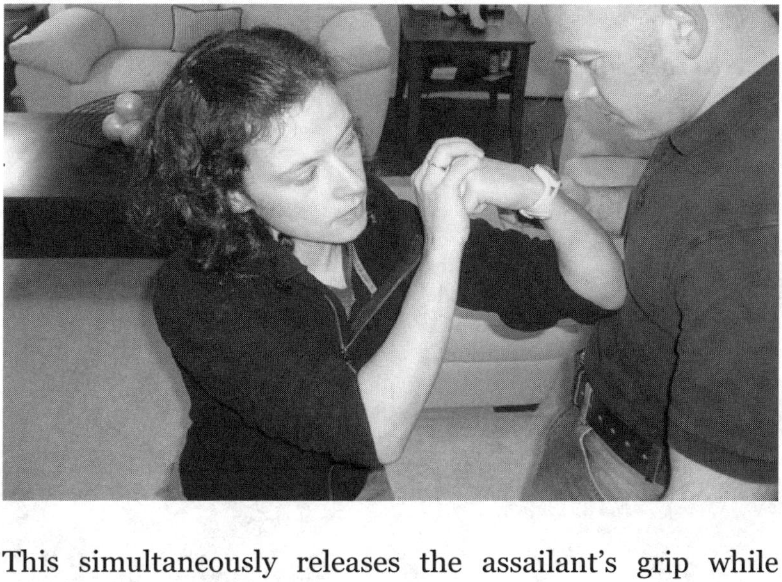

This simultaneously releases the assailant's grip while forcing the assailant away from you.

#3: One-handed lapel grab

This technique can be used to disengage from an assailant who has grabbed your lapel with one hand.

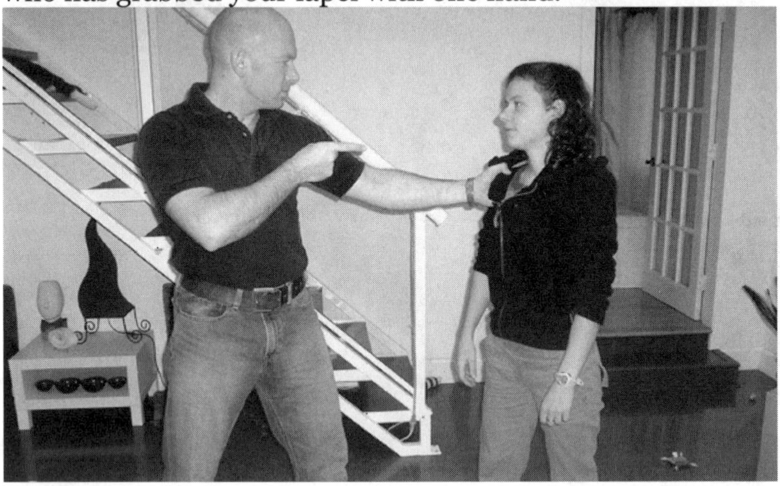

First, reach across your body with the hand on the opposite side to the side that the assailant is holding you. Grasp the assailant's hand firmly...

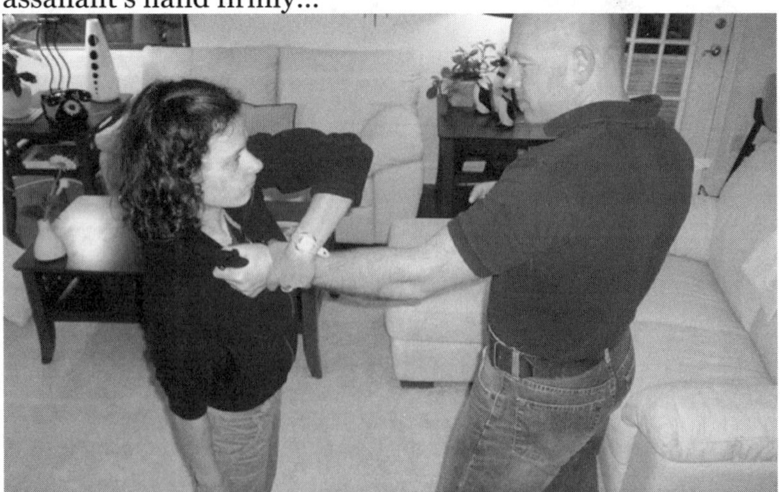

Maintaining the grip on the assailant's hand, swing your other hand up and drive it against the back of the assailant's elbow.

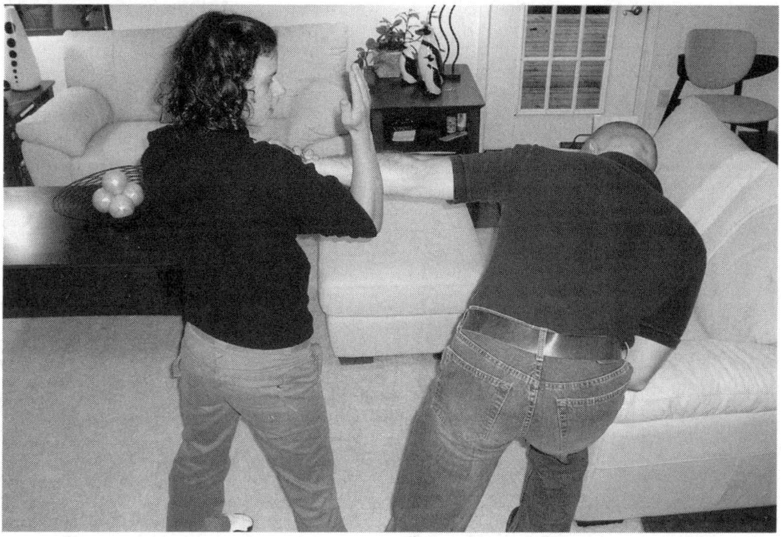

This locks the assailants elbow joint and wrist joint at the same time, forcing the assailant away from you.

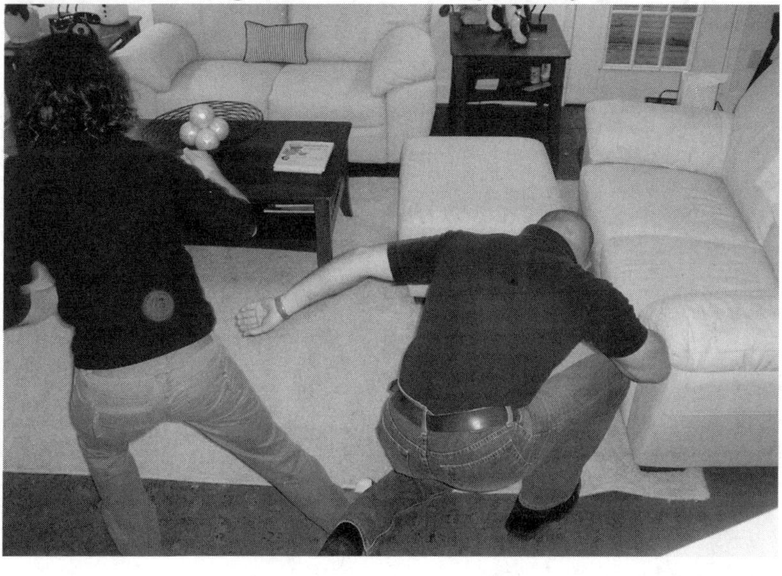

A variation on this is to grasp the assailant's hand with both of your hands...

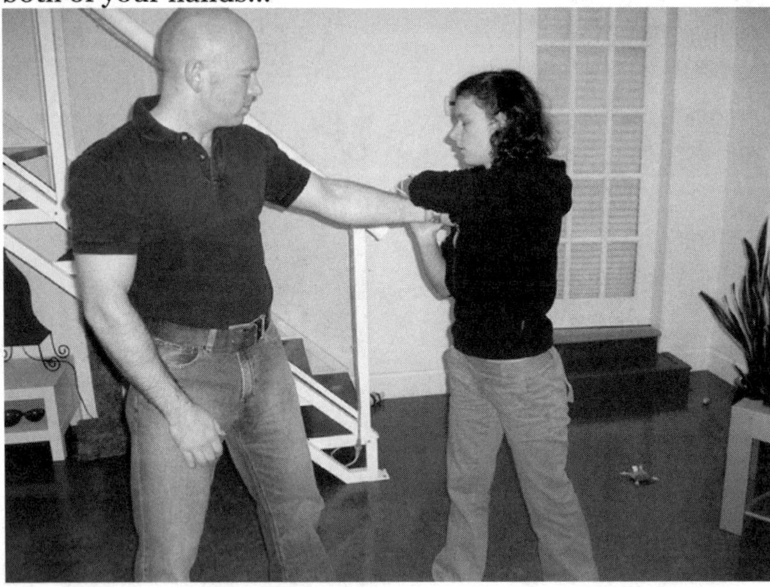

Then twist the assailant's wrist, locking his wrist...

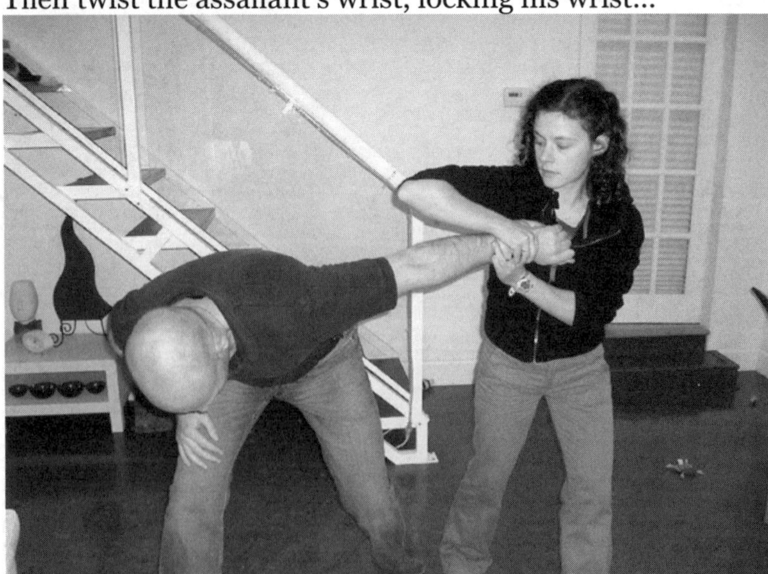

and forcing him away from you.

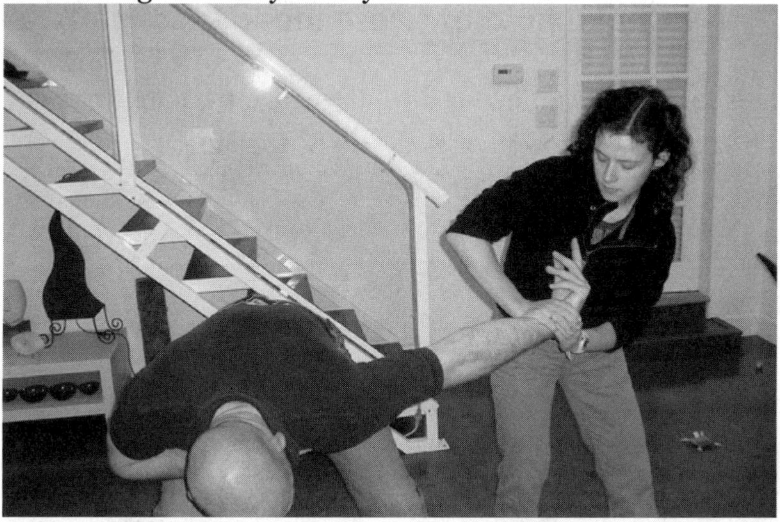

This procedure is simply reversed for a left-handed grab.

#4: Choke hold or two-handed lapel grab

This technique can be used to disengage from an assailant who tries to choke you or grab you by the lapels.

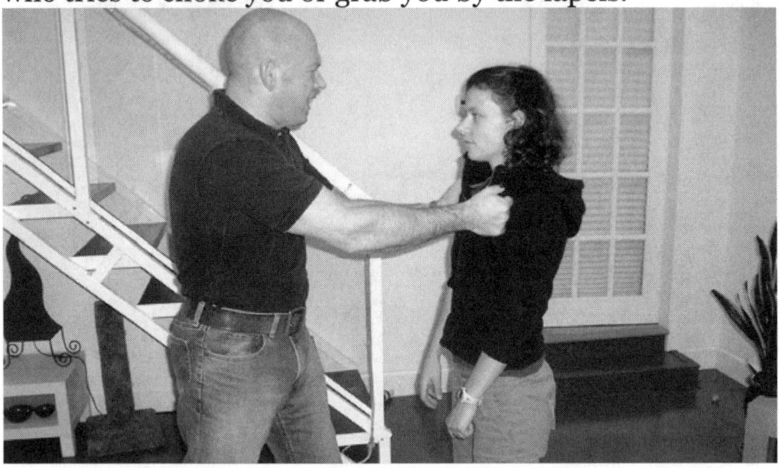

It is almost identical to the previous technique for dealing with a one-handed lapel grab. First reach across your body with either arm and grasp the assailant's wrist...

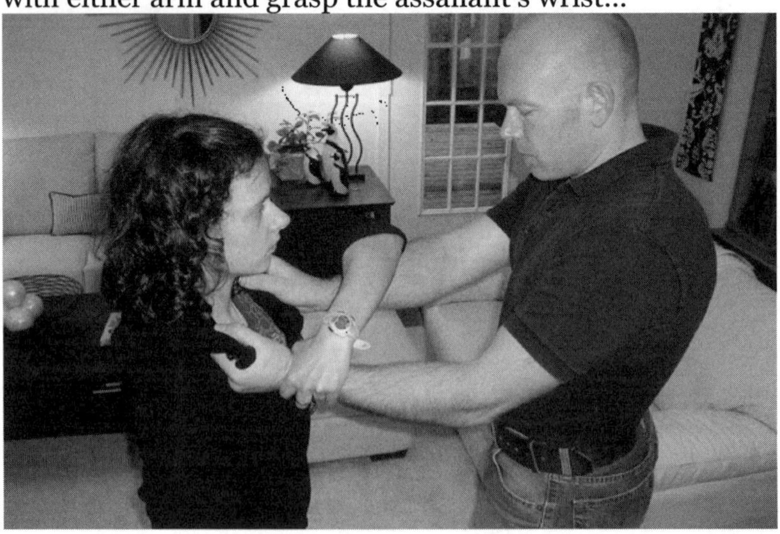

Maintaining the grip on the assailant's hand, swing your other hand up and drive it against the back of the assailant's elbow...

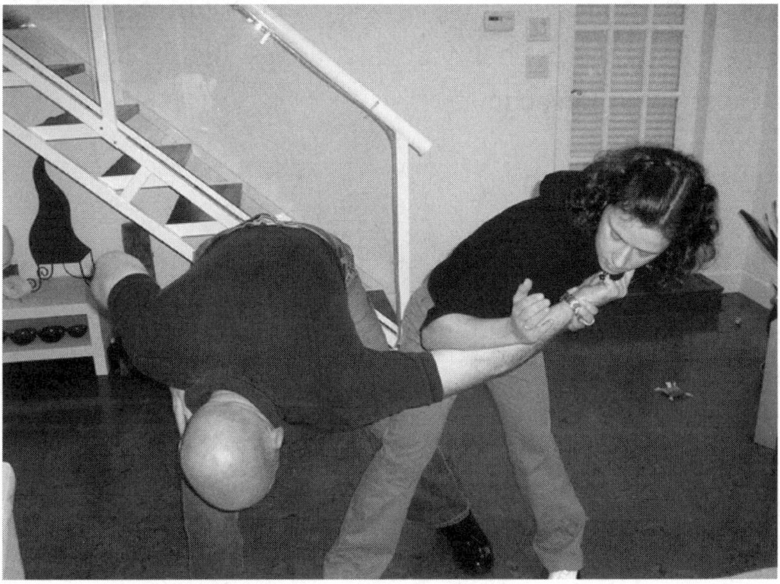

This locks the assailants elbow joint and wrist joint at the same time, forcing the assailant away from you.

#5: Bear hug:

This technique is used to disengage yourself from someone who comes up behind you and wraps his or her arms around your midsection.

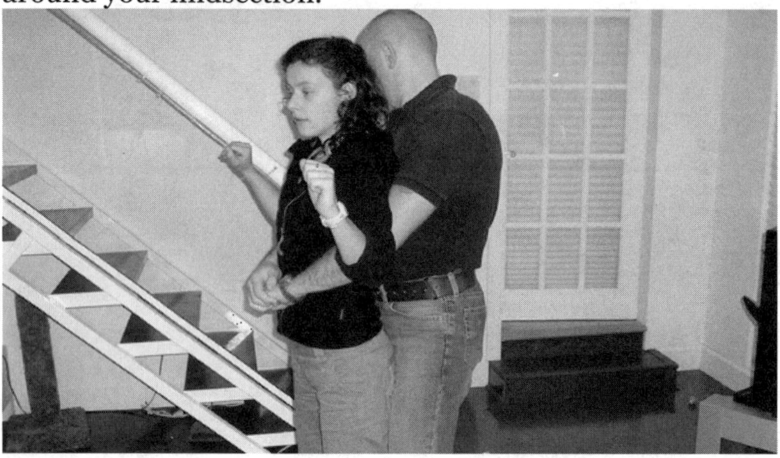

First, lower your center of gravity by taking a wide stance with your legs and squatting down slightly...

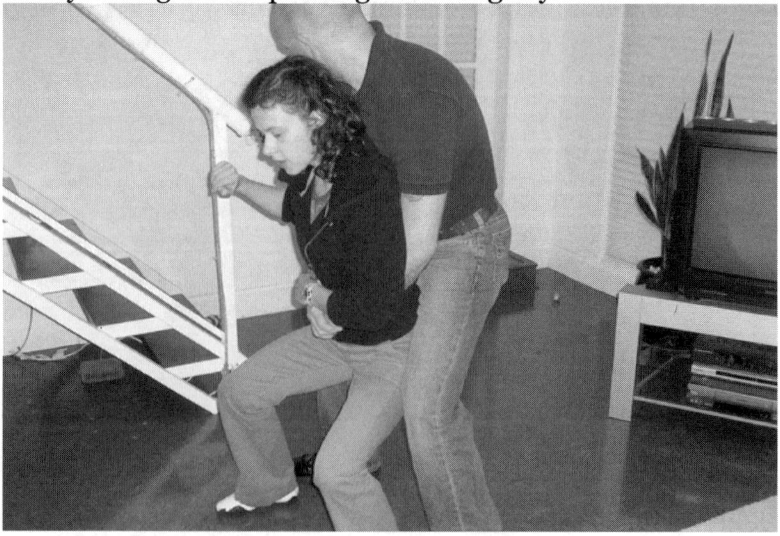

Reach across your abdomen with one arm and grasp one of the assailant's wrists. Hold on tightly...

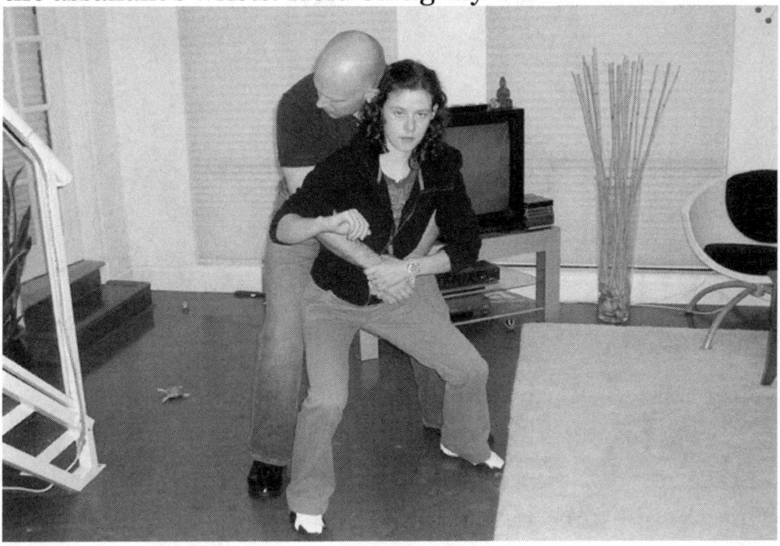

Twist to the other side rapidly, using your other arm to drive the assailant's head back...

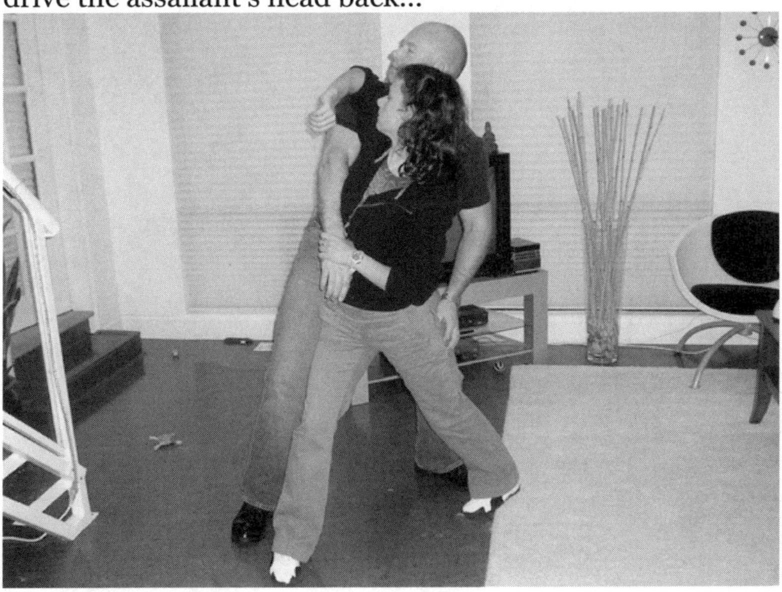

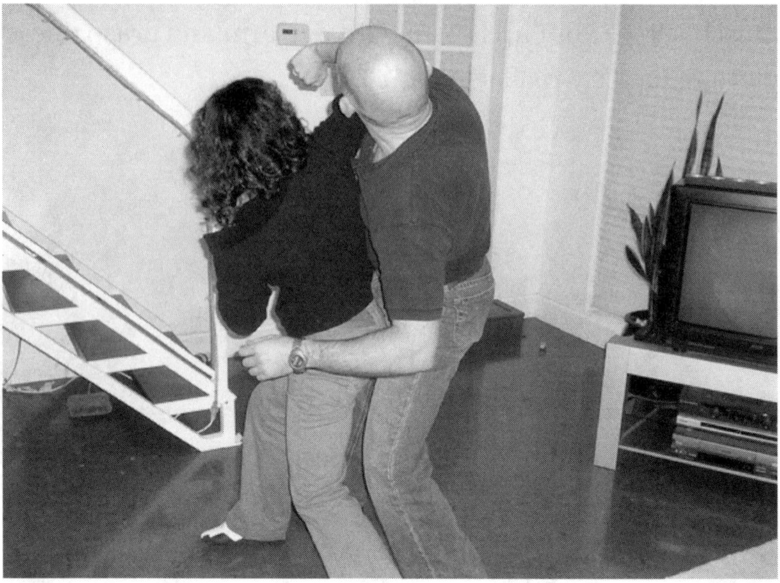

This should force the assailant to let go and knock him or her off balance, perhaps causing the assailant to fall to the ground.

#6: Head lock

This technique is used to disengage from an assailant who attempts to restrain you using a one-arm chokehold or headlock.

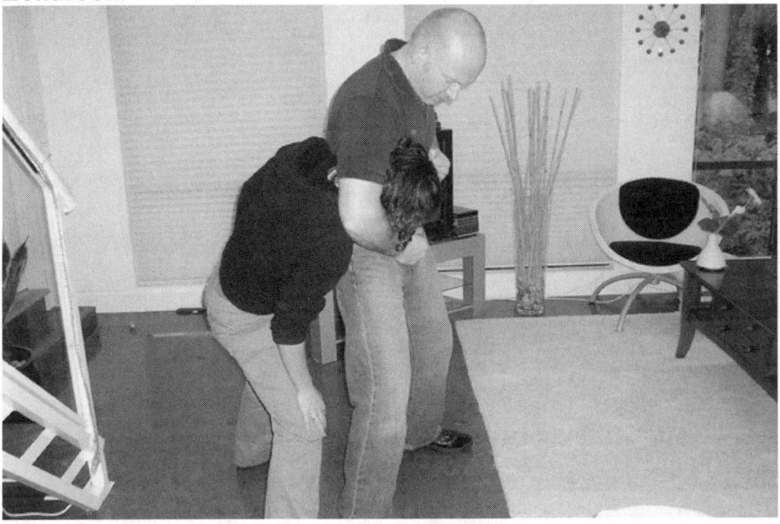

First, take a wide stance to give yourself stability...

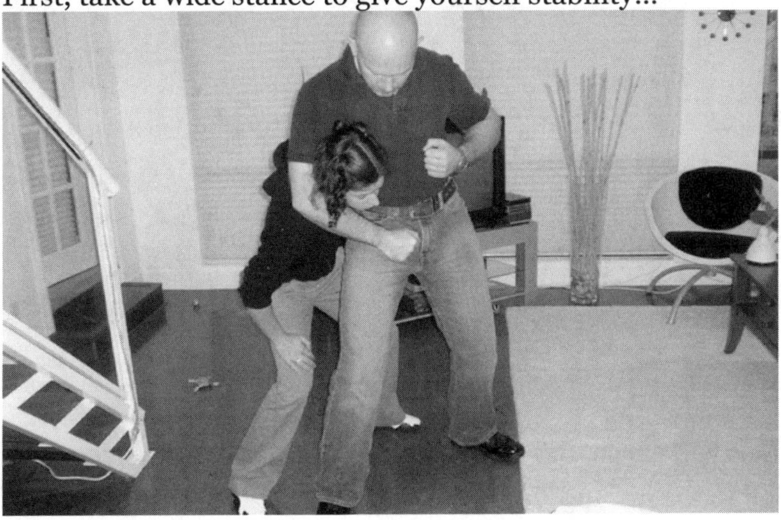

With the arm nearest your assailant, reach up over the assailant's shoulder. Put your hand under your assailant's chin and force your assailant's head back. With the other hand, grab under the assailant's leg closest to you and lift...

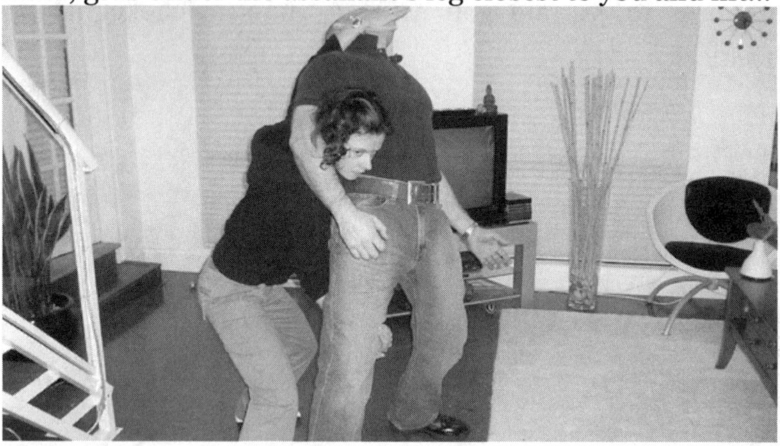

Stand up while continuing to force the assailant's head back and lifting the assailant's nearest leg...

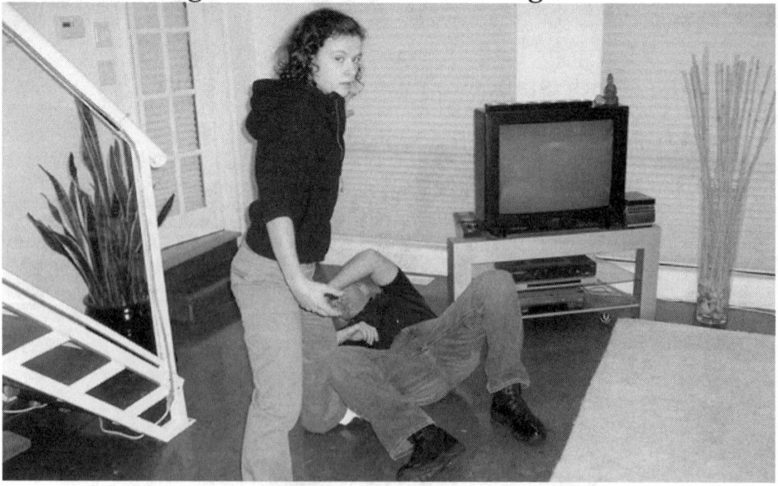

This will cause him to release his grip, lose his balance, and fall to the ground.

#7: Hair grab:

This technique can be used to disengage from an assailant who grabs you by the hair.

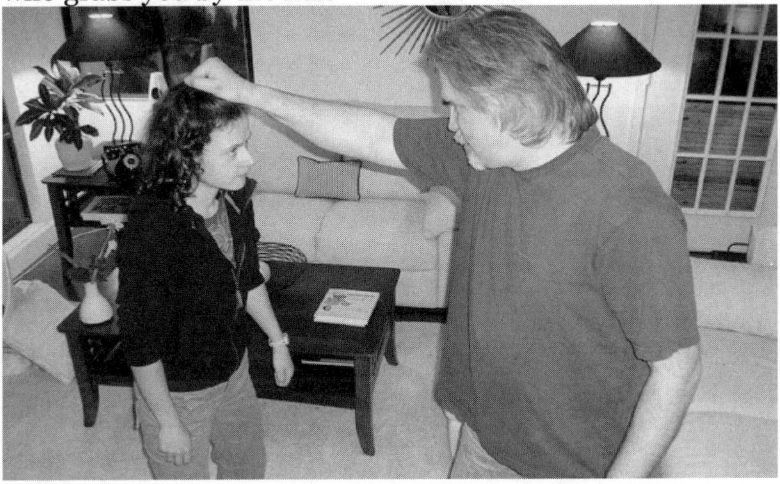

This is a variation of the technique we showed you earlier for disengaging from a one-handed lapel grab. First, with one hand, grab the hand that is holding you by the hair. Hold on tight...

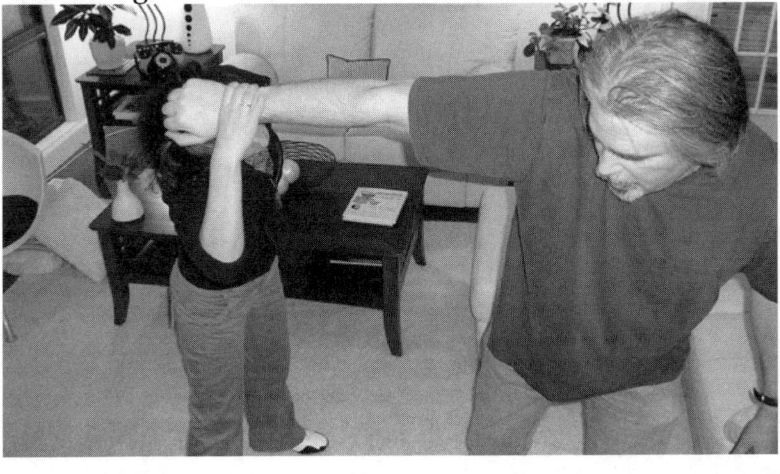

Next, twist the assailant's wrist while driving your other hand into the back of your assailant's elbow.

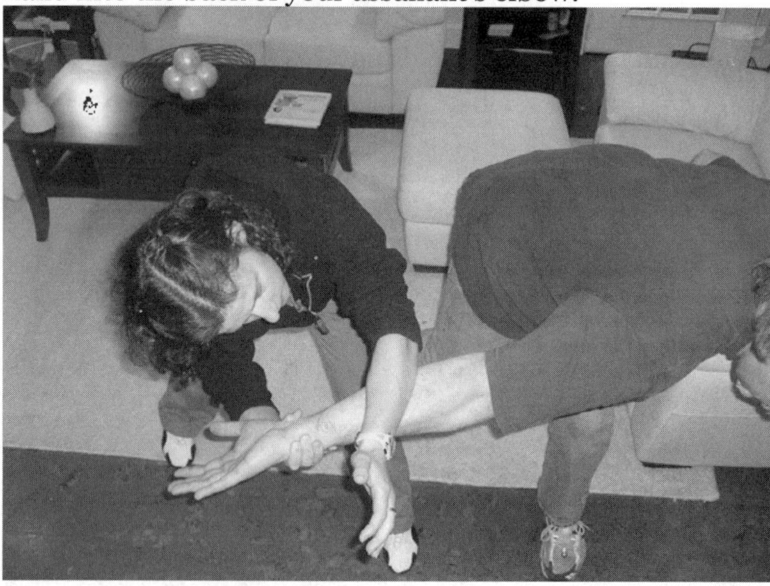

This will simultaneously lock the assailant's wrist and elbow and allow you to force him away from you.

Bibliography

BOOKS:

Adams, Ronald J., McTernan, Thomas M. & Remsberg, Charles. (1980). *Street survival: Tactics For armed encounters.* Evanston, IL: Calibre Press.

Adams, Ronald J., McTernan, Thomas M. & Remsberg, Charles. (1980). *Street survival seminar handout supplement.* Evanston, IL: Calibre Press.

Besharov, Douglas J. (1990). *Combating child abuse. Guidelines for cooperation between law enforcement and child protective services.* Washington, DC: The AEI Press.

Bibby, Pauline. (1994). *Personal safety for social workers.* Aldershot, Hants, UK: Arena Ashgate Publishing Ltd.

Brown, Robert, Bute, Stanley, & Ford, Peter. (1986). *Social workers at risk: The prevention and management of violence.* Basingstoke, Hampshire: Macmillan Education Ltd.

Greenwood, Supt. Colin. (1979). *Police tactics in armed operations.* Boulder, CO: Paladin Press.

Gregoire, Christine O. (February 1996). *Workplace security guide.* Olympia, WA: State of Washington, Office of the Attorney General.

Griffin, William V., Montsinger, James & Carter, Nancy. (1995). *Personal safety handbook: Targeting safety in human services.* Durham, NC: Brendan Associates.

Lalonde, Mark. (May 1997). *Safe at work: Strategies for preventing workplace violence in school settings.* New Westminster, BC: Justice Institute of British Columbia.

Morris, Jack. (1981). *The deadly routine.* Boulder, CO: Paladin Press.

Norris, Dan. (1990). *Violence against social workers: The implications for practice.* London: Jessica Kingsley Publishers.

Rowett, Colin. (1986). *Violence in social work: A research study of violence in the context of local authority social work.* Cambridge, UK: University of Cambridge.

United States Department of Labor, Occupational Safety and Health Administration. (1996). *Guidelines for preventing workplace violence for health care and social service workers.* OSHA 3148-1996.

ARTICLES:

Blauer, Tony. (Jan/Feb 1997) The theory of presumed compliance. *The Law Enforcement Trainer, 12*(1), 5-7.

Dillon, S. (1992, November 18). Social workers: Targets in a violent society. *The New York Times*, B6.

Griffin, William V. (1997). Staff safety in human services agencies. Protecting Children, 12(4), 13(1).

Harman, Patricia & Davis, Molly. (1997). Personal safety for human services professionals: A law enforcement perspective. *Protecting Children, 12*(4), 13(1).

Horejsi, Charles & Garthwait, Cindy. (1997). Be careful out there: CPS worker safety in rural areas. *Protecting Children, 12*(4), 13(1).

Irwin, Diane. (1997). Safety training for human services professionals. *Protecting Children, 12*(4), 13(1).

Kaplan, S. G. & Wheeler, E. G. (1983). Survival skills for working with potentially violent clients. *Social Casework, 64*, 339-346.

Lindsey, Bob. (Nov/ Dec 1996). Escalation and de-escalation of force. *The Law Enforcement Trainer, 11*(5), 9-11.

National Resource Center on Child Abuse and Neglect. (1997). Agency liability and worker safety. *Protecting Children, 12*(4), 13(1).

Rey, Lucy D. (1996). What social workers need to know about client violence. *Families in Society: The Journal of Contemporary Human Services, 77*(1).

Scalera, Nicholas R. (1995). The critical need for specialized health and safety measures for child welfare workers. *Child Welfare, 74*(2).

Schwarz, Victor. (1987). Social worker heal thyself. *Community Care*, 8 January.

Skiba, Janet T. & Cosner, Robert E. (Fall 1990). In harms way: A study of client assaults on Pennsylvania children and youth workers. *Pennsylvania Child Advocate Protective Services Quarterly, 5*(4).

Taylor, Douglas. (November 1996). How much OC is enough? *Law and Order, 44*(11), 27- 28.

VIDEOS:

Thompson, George J. (1992). *Verbal judo: The martial art of mind and mouth.* 3 part series. Jacksonville, FL: Institute of Police Technology and Management.

Notes

1 Dillon, S. (1992, November 18). Social workers: targets in a violent society. *New York Times*, p.1, B6.
2 National Clearinghouse on Child Abuse and Neglect Information. 2004. *Child abuse and neglect fatalities: Statistics and interventions.*
3 Ibid.
4 Newhill (1995), as cited in Shields, G. & Kiser, J. (2003). Violence and aggression directed toward human service workers: An exploratory study. *Families in Society, 84*(1), 14.
5 Stanley, J., and Goddard, C. (2002). *In the firing line*. England: Wiley & Sons, p. 119.
6 Ibid, p. 151.
7 Newhill, C. (1995). Client violence toward social workers: A practice and policy concern for the 1990's. *Social Work, 40*(5), 633.
8 Rowett, Colin. (1986). *Violence in social work: A research study of violence in the context of local authority social work*. Cambridge, England: University Of Cambridge.
9 Ibid, p 27.
10 Bibby, Pauline. (1994). *Personal safety for social workers.* Brookfield, VT: Ashgate Publishing. p. 17.
11 Sygnatur, Eric. F. & Toscano, Guy A. (2000). *Work related homicides: The facts*. Office of Safety, Health and Working Conditions, Bureau of Labor Statistics.
12 National Institute for Occupational Safety and Health (NIOSH). (2000). *Traumatic occupational injuries: Occupational violence.* http://www.cdc.gov/niosh/injury/traumaviolence.html
13 Gregoire, Christine O. (February 1996). *Workplace security guide.* State of Washington, Office of the Attorney General, p. 3.
14 Brown, Robert, Bute, Stanley, & Ford, Peter. (1986). *Social workers at risk: The prevention and management of violence*. Basingstoke, Hamps: Macmillan Education.
15 Ibid.
16 Ibid.
17 Bibby, Pauline. (1994). *Personal safety for social workers*. Fraser, MI: Arena. p. 12.
18 Ibid.

19 Ibid, p. 18.
20 Ibid.
21 Ibid, p. 13.
22 Jayaratne, Srinika, Croxton, Tom, & Mattison, Debra. (2004). A national survey of violence in the practice of social work. *Families in Society, 85*(4, Oct/Dec 2004):449.
23 Ibid, p 451.
24 Ibid, p.446.
25 Ibid, p. 451.
26 Astor, Ron Avi, Behre, William, Wallace, John M., & Fravil, Kimberely A. (May 1998). School social workers and school violence: Personal safety, training, and violence programs. *Social Work: Journal of the National Association of Social Workers, 43*(3):226.
27 Ibid.
28 Ibid, p 227.
29 Ibid, p 230.
30 Ibid.
31 Ibid.
32 Newhill, C. (1995). Client violence toward social workers: A practice and policy concern for the 1990's. *Social Work, 40*(5): 632.
33 Dillan, 1992, as cited in Newhill, 1995, p. 632.
34 Ibid.
35 Newhill, C. (October 1996). Prevalence and risk factors for client violence toward social workers. *Families in Society*, p. 491.
36 Jayaratne, Srinika; Croxton, Tom, and Mattison, Debra. (2004). A national survey of violence in the practice of social work. *Families in Society, 85*(4, Oct/Dec 2004): 445.
37 Ibid, p 447.
38 Ibid, p 449.
39 Ibid, p 452.
40 Gregoire, Christine O. (February 1996). *Workplace security guide.* State of Washington, Office of the Attorney General, p. 4.
41 Stanley, J., and Goddard, C. (2002). *In the firing line*. London, England: Wiley & Sons, p. 119.
42 Ibid, p 131.
43 Bibby, Pauline. (1994). *Personal safety for social workers*. p. 9.
44 MacDonald, G., & Sirotich, F. (2001). Reporting client violence. *Social Work, 46*(2): 107.
45 Scalera, Nicholas R. The critical need for specialized health and safety measures for child welfare workers. *Child Welfare, 74*(2): 339.
46 Harman, Patricia & Davis, Molly. (1997). Personal safety for human services professionals: A law enforcement perspective. *Protecting Children, 12*(4), & *13*(1).
47 Rowett, Colin. (1986). *Violence in social work.*
48 Schwarz, Victor. (1997, 8 January). Social worker heal thyself. *Community Care*, pp. 14-15.
49 Bibby, Pauline. (1994). *Personal safety for social workers*. p. 19.

50 Adams, Ronald J., McTernan, Thomas, & Remsberg, Charles. (1980). *Street survival: Tactics for armed encounters*. Northbrook, IL: Calibre Press. p. 42.
51 Rey, Lucy D. (January 1996). What social workers need to know about client violence. *Families in Society, The Journal of Contemporary Human Services, 77*(1): 36.
52 Bibby, Pauline. (1994). *Personal safety for social workers*. p. 8.
53 MacDonald, G., & Sirotich, F. (2001). Reporting client violence, *Social Work, 46*(2), p 112.
54 Ibid.
55 Ibid, p. 30.
56 Ibid, p. 31.
57 Rowett, Colin. (1986). *Violence in social work*.
58 Leadbetter, 1993, as cited in MacDonald, G., & Sirotich, F. (2001). Reporting client violence. *Social Work, 46*(2): 109.
59 MacDonald, G., & Sirotich, F. (2001). Reporting client violence. *Social Work, 46*(2): 111.
60 Ibid.
61 Ibid, p 113.
62 Cited in Shields, G. & Kiser, J. (2003). Violence and aggression directed toward human service workers: An exploratory study. *Families in Society, 84*(1): 14.
63 United States Department of Labor, Occupational Safety and Health Administration. (1996). *Guidelines for preventing workplace violence for health care & social service workers*. OSHA 3148-1996, p 9.
64 Skiba, Janet T. and Cosner, Robert E. (Fall 1990). In harms way: A study of client assaults on Pennsylvania children and youth workers. *Pennsylvania Child Advocate and Protective Services Quarterly, 5*(4), 6.
65 Newhill, C. (1995). Client violence toward social workers: A practice and policy concern for the 1990's. *Social Work, 40*(5), 633.
66 Ibid, p 635.
67 Kaplan, S. G. & Wheeler, E.G. (1983). Survival skills for working with potentially violent clients. *Social Casework, 64*, 339.
68 Rowett, Colin. (1986). *Violence in social work*. p. 27.
69 Brown, Robert, Bute, Stanley, and Ford, Peter. (1986). *Social workers at risk*.
70 Ibid.
71 Brown, Robert, Bute, Stanley, and Ford, Peter. (1986). *Social workers at risk*.
72 Gregoire, Christine O. (February 1996). *Workplace security guide*. State of Washington, Office of the Attorney General, p. 4.
73 Brown, Robert, Bute, Stanley, and Ford, Peter. (1986). *Social workers at risk*.
74 British Columbia Ministry of Children and Families statistics, 1995/96.
75 Brown, Robert, Bute, Stanley, and Ford, Peter. (1986). *Social workers at risk*.

76 Adams, Ronald J., McTernan, Thomas, and Remsberg, Charles. (1980). *Street survival: Tactics for armed encounters*. Northbrook, IL: Caliber Press, p. 35.
77 Bibby, Pauline. (1994). *Personal safety for social workers*. p. 9.
78 Ibid., p. 8.
79 Ibid., p 9.
80 Ibid.
81 New York City Police Department. (1974). *Analysis of police combat situations*.
82 Adapted from: Adams, Ronald J., McTernan, Thomas, and Remsberg, Charles. (1980). *Street survival: Tactics for armed encounters*, p. 6.
83 Rowett, Colin. (1986). *Violence in social work*. p. 6.
84 Ibid.
85 Brown, Robert, Bute, Stanley, and Ford, Peter. (1986). *Social workers at risk*.
86 Ibid., pp. 30-31.
87 Rowett, Colin. (1986). *Violence in social work*. p. 135.
88 Adams, Ronald J., McTernan, Thomas M. and Remsberg, Charles. (1980). *Street survival seminar handout supplement*.
89 Blauer, Tony. (January/February 1997). The theory of presumed compliance. *The Law Enforcement Trainer, 12*(1), 6.
90 Ibid.
91 Skiba, Janet T. and Cosner, Robert E. (Fall 1990). In harms way: A study of client assaults on Pennsylvania children and youth workers. *Pennsylvania Child Advocate and Protective Services Quarterly, 5*(4), 8.
92 Blau, P. M. & Scott, W. R. (1962). *Formal organizations: A comparative approach*. San Francisco, CA: Chandler Publishing. p. 27.
93 Ibid. p 28.
94 Ibid.
95 Bibby, Pauline. (1994). *Personal safety for social workers*. p. 131.
96 Star (1984) as cited in Skiba, Janet T. and Cosner, Robert E. (Fall 1990). In harms way: A study of client assaults on Pennsylvania children and youth workers. *Pennsylvania Child Advocate and Protective Services Quarterly, 5*(4), 4.
97 Ibid.
98 Adams, Ronald J., McTernan, Thomas, and Remsberg, Charles. (1980). *Street survival: tactics for armed encounters*, pp. 30-31.
99 Rowett, Colin. (1986). *Violence in social work*. p. 92.
100 Lindsey, Bob. (January/February 1999). Learning from the American tragedy: The wounding and killing of law enforcement officers in the United States, Part Three: Back to basics. *The Law Enforcement Trainer, 14*(1), p 9.
101 Scalera, Nicholas R. The critical need for specialized health and safety measures for child welfare workers. *Child Welfare, 74*(2), 339.

102 Horejsi, Charles and Garthwaite, Cindy. (1997). Be careful out there: CPS worker safety in rural areas. *Protecting Children, 12*(4), 13(1).
103 Ibid.
104 Besharov, Douglas J. (1990). *Combating child abuse: Guidelines for cooperation between law enforcement and child protective services*. p 27.
105 Skiba, Janet T. and Cosner, Robert E. (Fall 1990). In harms way: A study of client assaults on Pennsylvania children and youth workers. *Pennsylvania Child Advocate and Protective Services Quarterly, 5*(4), 2.
106 Thompson, George J., PhD. (1992). Verbal judo: *The martial art of mind and mouth* (3 part video series).
107 Ibid.
108 Lindsey, Bob. (November/December 1996). Escalation and de-escalation of force. *The Law Enforcement Trainer, 11*(5), 10.
109 Skiba, Janet T. and Cosner, Robert E. (Fall 1990). In harms way: A study of client assaults on Pennsylvania children and youth workers. *Pennsylvania Child Advocate and Protective Services Quarterly, 5*(4), 3.
110 Horejsi, Charles and Garthwaite, Cindy. (1997). Be careful out there: CPS worker safety in rural areas. *Protecting Children, 12*(4), 13(1).
111 Adams, Ronald J., McTernan, Thomas M. and Remsberg, Charles. (1980). *Street survival seminar handout supplement*.
112 BCGEU submission to the Royal Commission on Worker's Compensation in British Columbia, July 1997, p 32.

Index

About the Authors

Charles Ennis retired after a 29-year career with the Vancouver Police Department and is now a police dispatcher. Ennis worked with Child Protection Workers and Psychiatric Nurses in the field from May 1996 until his retirement in 2005. He was a member of the Emergency Response Team Tactical Unit and a Gang Crime Unit investigator for many years. Ennis is a published author and safety trainer for police, social workers, and nurses.

Janet Douglas has been a frontline child protection social worker in Vancouver, B.C. for the past 21 years, working with families in crisis. She has worked for over a decade in a specialized emergency response unit with the Vancouver Police, where she and her co-author investigated high-risk child abuse complaints where there were concerns about the potential for violence. The authors have trained numerous agencies and their staff on how to be safe when working in the field. Janet Douglas has both a Bachelor's and Master's degree in social work, and is currently working on her Ph.D.